30

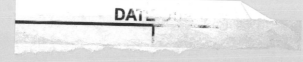

Autism and its Medical Management

of related interest

Autism Heroes
Portraits of Families Meeting the Challenge
Barbara Firestone, Ph.D.
Forewords by Teddi Cole and Gary Cole and Catherine Lord, Ph.D.
Photographs by Joe Buissink
ISBN 978 1 84310 837 5

New Developments in Autism
The Future is Today
Edited by Juan Martos Pérez, Pedro M. González, María Llorente Comí and Carmen Nieto
ISBN 978 1 84310 449 0

Everyday Education
Visual Support for Children with Autism
Pernille Dyrbjerg and Maria Vedel
Foreword by Lennart Pedersen
ISBN 978 1 84310 457 5

The Development of Autism
A Self-Regulatory Perspective
Thomas L. Whitman
ISBN 978 1 84310 735 4

Understanding the Nature of Autism and Asperger's Disorder
Forty Years of Clinical Practice and Pioneering Research
Edward R. Ritvo, M.D., Professor Emeritus, UCLA School of Medicine
Foreword by Tony Attwood
ISBN 978 1 84310 814 6

Autism and its Medical Management

A Guide for Parents and Professionals

Michael G. Chez MD

Jessica Kingsley Publishers
London and Philadelphia

First published in 2008
by Jessica Kingsley Publishers
116 Pentonville Road
London N1 9JB, UK
and
400 Market Street, Suite 400
Philadelphia, PA 19106, USA

www.jkp.com

Copyright © Michael G. Chez 2008

Library of Congress Cataloging in Publication Data
A CIP catalog record for this book is available from the Library of Congress

British Library Cataloguing in Publication Data
A CIP catalogue record for this book is available from the British Library

ISBN 978 1 84310 834 4

Printed and bound in the United States by
Thomson-Shore, Inc.

This book is dedicated to my immediate family: my wife Dawn, who has always believed in my abilities to help children with disabilities, and my children, Rebecca, Ariel, Colleen, and Alison, who have been an important part of my becoming a better human being, and father, and therefore a better doctor. I am indebted to my office staff who have helped me through the years, and to my patients, their parents and families, and to all who have believed in me over the course of caring for those with neurological conditions that sought my care. I am thankful that I continue to have the desire to always learn ways to be better at my profession.

Special thanks to Tim Dowling, Laura Wald, Mina Chang, Dawn Chez, Robert Hughes, Rudy and Marcy Valner, the Ward family, Shawna Egan, and many others who helped make suggestions and offered support during the writing of this book. I thank Jessica Kingsley Publishers for giving me the opportunity to write this book.

Finally, I dedicate this book to my colleagues in medicine who, despite the frustrations and sometimes slow progress associated with trying to help children with developmental delays, continue to make new discoveries every day.

Contents

List of Tables

List of Figures

Preface

In the past 60 years, autistic behaviors have been medically described. The behaviors were officially first termed "autism" by psychiatrist Leo Kanner at Johns Hopkins Hospital in 1943, and much observational research has been done by subsequent psychologists and psychiatrists. Despite fairly universal agreement corresponding to a core of behavioral symptoms that label a child at risk for these autistic spectrum conditions, no single theory as to the cause of these behaviors has yet evolved and been proven. Once thought a rare condition, it now appears that autistic spectrum disorders are now the leading cause of childhood developmental disorders. The frequency may be greater than 1:150 births. Despite these numbers of cases, there is still debate among medical professionals whether this condition is increasing or just becoming more recognized. Complicating the definition of autism is that many medical conditions that can damage the brains of developing infants can overlap autistic spectrum disorders. Despite increasing research efforts, the exact localization for autistic behavior, and the exact neuroanatomical or biochemical mechanisms that cause the condition, remains a mystery to be solved. Many authors have written about autism, and in their pioneering book, *The Biology of the Autistic Syndromes*, Coleman and Gillberg aptly coined the term "autistic syndromes." I plan to use this idea of subtyping characteristics of the spectrum disorder of autism to practically describe treatment strategies in this book. This may differ from strict definitions of the DSM-IV-TR, where all autistic conditions are under the umbrella of pervasive developmental disorders. I will refer to the autistic spectrum disorders through the rest of this book as ASD, and where necessary refer to the separate categories of autism (the pervasive developmental disorders will be PDD) and Asperger's syndrome as unique entities as well. I will also discuss clinically observed subtypes of autism, such as autism caused by extreme prematurity, birth injury, chronic epilepsy, or genetic disorders. I will refer to traditional aspects of this condition simply as autism.

There is no current cure for autism. A sad observation that I have made is the lack of training in the pediatric community for children with autism, and the confusion and fear that overtakes parents because medical professionals have been somewhat unprepared for the impact this childhood condition manifests both for the child and the parents. This has created poor communication at times between pediatricians and child specialists and the families of autistic children. Sometimes this is based upon stereotypes and the lack of physician training in the latest facts and theories of autism as a neurological condition whose symptoms have medical treatment options, even if autism at this time remains incurable. For parents there is often a fear that their doctor may offer them no help, or that remnants of the out-of-date theory of the "refrigerator parent" model from the 1950s will blame them for causing their child's problems. Unfortunately, this theory was psychoanalytically promoted by psychiatrists such as Bruno Bettelheim, who blamed the cause of autism on aloof mothers who were distant emotionally from their infants. This has created anger among some advocacy groups for autism and caused mistrust of traditional medicine. A legacy of fringe medicine masquerading as science, leading parents to poor care and often expensive quackery that has not really benefited any significant number of sufferers, has therefore offered parents more hope than well-trained neurologists and psychiatrists. I hope this book can elevate parental understanding of the complexity of autism, yet arm families and professionals with a common sense approach to this developmental condition of childhood.

Autistic disorders do not usually shorten expected lifespan, so we need to prepare for long-term care of these children as they grow to adulthood. Everyone will be directly or indirectly affected by the economic burden autism spectrum disorders will place on our society. Staggering costs of 3.5 million dollars per affected child are estimated to be the direct cost of caring for an autistic individual through their lifespan. Improving early intervention and quality of life, reversing some aspects of these autistic behaviors at a neurological level, and improving social deficits in communication and awareness of others will benefit everyone. I hope in the future to write updated editions of this book and be able to talk of treatments that may reverse or prevent autism.

As I complete this book, I thank all the patients and their families that have sought my care over the past 14 years. I entered the autism maze with little to guide me and often have felt as one of the "blind men describing an elephant." The trust and efforts of the families I have met have inspired me to look for new answers, and to open my mind to possible new treatments. I have also seen tragic false hopes and expensive treatments by so-called alternative practitioners, which sometimes, though thankfully rarely, have even endangered the safety of some of my patients. More commonly these misleading therapies have just caused disappointment and financial loss. My biggest disappointment is that early medical evaluation and treatment is often delayed. It also is my hope that this book will prevent these abuses that prey upon desperate parents, and hope that one day neurological scientific advances will define the exact etiology and treatment options for the various subtypes of autistic spectrum disorders. At this time the medical establishment is still organizing how to offer appropriate treatment by researching how to prove the effectiveness of medicines to be used. That does not mean that physicians have not been experiencing success using available medicines to relieve the physical and emotional symptoms for children and families with ASD.

This book is written for parents, interested lay people, therapists of various types, and also for physicians to give insight into what can actually be done today. I will give a bibliography with medical references at the end of the book. The majority of the book is meant to be more readable for both interested parents and professionals. Because the research is happening so fast that references for ASD may quickly be out of date, I humbly hope I have caught the majority of the latest and comprehensive important references. I have gleaned these facts for the medical chapters on the background, theories, and treatment portions of this book. Therefore, all the scientific discussion is based on actual medical facts that I have pulled from past historically important articles and today's breaking research papers. All the treatments discussed in this book have medical evidence as actually working in some way to help improve core symptoms or secondary problems with ASD derived from the medical literature available to physicians in the United States, as well as Europe, Israel, Eastern Europe, Asia, North America, South America, or Australia. Therefore, only medically based treatments with at least some published reference are offered as possible treatment choices for patients with ASD in the discussion in this book. Alternative or dietary treatments that have actual clinical research based publications are also explained as possibly effective. Treatments that are mythical, based on false theories, or have not shown truly meaningful clinical outcomes are pointed out as well. I purposely wrote the book this way as I do not expect parents of children with ASD always to be able to decipher medical research papers, and I fully expect physicians to be able to confirm the scientific facts by utilizing available medical research search technology on the topics discussed.

The ideas in this book, however, can serve as a clear guide to both groups in organizing a variety of potential treatment plans that medically can be used for a child with ASD when indicated by the specific clinical profiles. This book is not intended to be a cookbook for treatment. Any treatment for an individual must still be done between the actual patient and their treating physician.

Introduction and Reader Guide

This book is a work designed to help parents and professionals comprehend the vast options available for current treatment of problems that are medical in nature and associated with the condition most people refer to as "autism." It will hopefully be understood that since autism is a heterogeneous condition, that subtypes of this condition will naturally exist. This is why I like to refer to these differing subtypes as autistic spectrum disorders (ASD). Different treatments will affect different subtypes to varying degrees. Autism is a very complex medical condition; I will try to the best of my ability to discuss causation and treatment for the autism spectrum conditions as far as is known about them at the time of this publication. I honestly believe that this book may become out of date within a matter of a few years as I expect great progress in the near future of autism research.

The chapters are deliberately not written in the form of a traditional medical textbook. I wrote this book to be as readable as possible for physicians, parents, and non-medical professionals. This is not meant to be an encyclopedic edition on the medical care of autism, nor is it to serve as a "cookbook" for treatment. In no circumstance is this book anything more than suggestions and information on how I feel autism spectrum disorders may be medically treated to improve quality of life. This information is supported by the medical literature wherever possible, and reflects almost two decades of my own practice experience. This book is meant to serve as information to open dialogue for physicians and patients regarding the available medical treatment options for autism today. This required the chapters not to include references within the text; instead they are given in Appendix 1 for those interested in the facts in the medical literature.

As with all authors, I admit there may be author bias in some areas and that some material may be early and theoretical. I hope that I successfully and honestly have tried to note these points in the chapters as still being theoretical or based on my personal experience only. Also, I do not expect every reader fully to understand every technical point, especially in chapters on genetics, electroencephalography (EEG), neuroimaging, or immunology. I try to offer summation of pertinent points wherever possible as the take-home message.

I have not really included a chapter on speech therapy, occupational therapy, or developmental therapies for autism such as Dr. Greenspan's "Floortime" or Dr. Lovaas' applied behavioral therapy or "ABA," nor recent therapies such as augmented typing or rapid letter boards, or offshoots of behavioral therapies like relationship development intervention (RDI). I did this because as a child neurologist who focuses on medical diagnosis and treatment, I feel there is already a willingness among experts and the public to try these behavioral and support measures early in autism. There are already children referred to speech and occupational therapists at an early age through community-based early childhood intervention. The emphasis on this book is the medical arena, one that, in my opinion, gets currently relegated to the last step, with parents often delaying getting medical treatment for fear of the labeling of their child, or their own fear of how medications may affect their children physically. These myths and fears must be overcome, and I hope that this book will explain what is currently available for successful quality-of-life improvement for children and adults within the autism spectrum.

PART I
Autism Overview

Chapter 1

What Is Normal Development?

Does My Child Have Autism?

The first step in getting help is by recognizing that your child may have a problem. Defining autism clinically and how psychologists and physicians define the disorder are explained in the next two chapters. For parents and some primary care physicians, early recognition for children at risk is a critical first step. To begin with, earlier medical and therapy intervention has been shown to improve long-term outcome.

Children develop in well-understood stages through infancy and toddler years. The first thing to note is the newborn period. Did the child have any problems being born, or at the delivery? Low muscle tone, fetal distress, poor oral motor feeding, or excessive infant irritability are possible future risk factors. Another unusual story is the "too good" baby that never really demands attention from parents even in the first three months. Either extreme of "too good" or "terribly irritable" may suggest the infant is at risk for developmental problems. Infants are supposed to track and smile between four and six weeks of age. They like being held and cuddled. If these factors are absent by three months of age, let the pediatrician know. Motor development should follow a pattern of rolling over from front to back, and back to front by six months of age, sitting up between six and eight months, and pulling to a stand by 14 months. Crawling should occur by nine months to one year and should not come after walking. Walking should begin between 10 and 15 months in normal development.

Levels of alertness and normal awake and asleep cycles may also be indicators of development.

Speech development is critical to humans, and has both nonverbal and verbal components. The start of social communication is the way the infant tracks others or seeks to make eye contact in the first three months. The infant may then coo or make sounds and smile socially to the parents between two and four months of age. Interest in toys shown by batting or holding toys should begin no later than six months of age. Putting objects in the mouth is part of normal oral motor and speech development at between 6 and 18 months of age. Consonants and vowels begin at six months to one year, and "mama" or "dada" sounds present in most cultures by 12 months. Games such as "peek-a-boo" or "pat-a-cake," waving, pointing, and reaching to be picked up by a parent should begin by 15 months of age. Clues to oral motor problems may be early feeding problems, excessive drooling, poor tongue control, or choking excessively when fed. Any problems with these early communication steps should warrant attention. Subsequent speech usually shows rapid increases in word and phrase acquisition in the 12- to 24-month period. It becomes critical to monitor and track acquisition and appropriate use of new words. Any stagnation or loss of previusly acquired words or gestures suggests the child may be regressing or developing a speech or hearing problem.

This is an important time to monitor whether a child responds to verbal commands or communication. Children should turn when you call out their names and make eye contact. Any lack of interest in that area should be brought to your pediatrician's attention, especially if a change or loss of these skills occurs. Parents need to monitor these issues closely. These details may help define the difference between true regression in autistic spectrum disorders (ASD) and children who were always at risk and are just developing in an abnormal pattern.

Self-stimulatory gestures may occur in ASD. These may be unusual holding of toys, staring at lights, fingers, fans, swirling water or faucets, car wheels, or lining up of objects. Excessive fascination with letters, symbols, shapes, or numbers at less than 24 months of age is abnormal. Hand flapping, twirling, rocking, finger flicking, or stiffening and shuddering may be an autistic behavior, but remember some children at risk for Tourette's syndrome, anxiety, or up to 5 percent of normal children may exhibit some form of automatisms or self-stimulatory movements during development. Bringing these behaviors to the attention of your physician is important. Handedness is also important. If a child picks using the left or right hand exclusively before 15 months, there may be something wrong, such as a corresponding hemi-paralysis or stroke-like problem that may come from early brain injury. Later, after two years of age, if a child has not picked dominance of handedness, it may be a marker for motor planning delay, and often in ASD, children will have mixed hand dominance corresponding to their motor planning deficits.

Physicians should be told of the patterns described above, but they should also ask about these developmental traits. Children who are not speaking or making good social nonverbal effort by 12 to 15 months of age should be referred for neurological and auditory evaluation. It is not true that children should stop talking because they are boys, are just developing gross motor skills, or have a new sibling born. Early referral is so critical, and medical evaluation of possible neurodevelopmental problems should not be delayed. Table 1.1 shows normal skill acquisition summary.

Table 1.1 Normal developmental patterns in the first two years of life

Age (months)	Normal developmental stages—Motor
0–4	Pick up head, push up, may roll over
4–8	Roll over both ways, sit up, may bat toys, crawl
8–12	Crawl, pull up, take first steps, pincer grasp
12–24	Walk/run, use utensils to eat, roll a ball, stack blocks

Age (months)	Normal developmental stages—Nonverbal
0–3	Smile, track, hug or grasp
4–12	Mouth objects, reach out, turn when called
12–18	Good eye contact, follow commands: wave gesture and point, peek-a-boo, clap, imitate

Age (months)	Normal developmental stages—Verbal
0–6	"Coo," raspberry vowels
6–12	Consonants and vowels, combination sounds, first words: "Ma," "Da"
12–24	First words, increase vocabulary, intonation, single two-word phrases, 50 words by 18 months, 200–500 words age 24 months

If any child has delays in the normal social or communication realms by 12 to 15 months of age, the cause must be evaluated and parents should be aware the child may be at risk for ASD or some other neurological disorder. Parents and professionals should also identify children delayed in more than one area. For example, gross motor delays with communication delays is often representative of an underlying disorder like cerebral palsy, or genetic or metabolic deficits. Also unusual facial features, large head size and deformities of heart, genitals, kidneys, or skin may reflect an underlying chromosomal disorder. All these factors should cause parents to seek out appropriate medical care. For children who seem deaf or to have regressed in understanding words, an early hearing test should be obtained by 12 to 15 months of age.

In summary then, parents and medical care providers in infancy should be aware of normal social, language, and motor developmental milestones. Variation from normal should not be assumed to be acceptable. Early screening of parental concerns is critical to effective early interventional help, and appropriate referrals for diagnosis and treatment.

Chapter 2

Understanding the Diagnosis of Autism

Most of the common myths of autism started from misleading theories of the 1940s through the 1960s. From the beginning in the 1940s, Dr. Leo Kanner, a psychiatrist at Johns Hopkins Hospital, realized he was observing a unique medical entity. He also unfortunately assigned blame to the parents of children affected with autism. Roughly at the same time Dr. Asperger in Austria described similar behaviors among higher-functioning children. These men were working independently at the time. By the 1950s, psychological theories went even further, blaming mothers for causing the lack of emotional bonding of their autistic children. In addition to the psychological aspects, Dr. Kanner failed by modern standards to define subtle neurological criteria, and of course he did not have access to current chromosomal, metabolic, or neuroimaging or electrophysiological studies. Despite this lack of modern technology, even Kanner noted the presence of seizures and abnormal electroencephalograms (EEG) in some of his original 11 autistic patients even during the 1940s. These observations were among the first showing that the biological aspects of this disability were undeniable.

Despite availability of improved medical diagnostic tests over the past half century, a common causative factor for children affected with autistic behaviors still eludes physicians. Psychologists have standardized testing for differentiating autism from pervasive developmental disorder (PDD) or mental retardation, but practically for physicians, these distinctions are not biologically meaningful. Parents are often misled by the confusing terminology, and are given different descriptive or diagnostic labels for their children by occupational therapists, speech therapists, or educational specialists—such as sensory integration disorder, aphasia, apraxia, nonverbal learning disability, or other descriptive terminology. Therefore all the terms used for autistic spectrum disorders (ASD) rely upon description, not biological definition. At the present time, very few parents initially think to ask for medical causes to their child's condition, and often avoid looking for serious medical or chronic neurological causes for these clinical issues. This is partially the fault of denial, and also the lack of education among general pediatricians to refer for a neurological evaluation of most children early in their 12- to 24-month development. Sometimes this is because parents and pediatricians want more time to observe. The negative result of this pattern of first referring to speech or occupational therapists, psychologists, or school systems is that it delays early diagnostic medical intervention. In addition, traditional medicine has not been very helpful in autism in the past, offering little in the research or education about the biology of this condition, and often sending parents away feeling there is little to be done or hoped for. This possibility of parents facing a chronic health condition in their toddler with no hope of medical help has led to desperate alternative therapies that mostly do nothing to help these children.

Therefore, for most parents and professionals, there has been erected a stigma of labeling very young children with autism. When confronted with worrisome behavior in a young child, many professionals, especially pediatricians in the United States, are uncomfortable telling young families that their child may have autism. Often this is referred to as not using the "A-Word." The terms pervasive developmental disorder or sensory integration disorder have been erroneously used to describe potentially autistic children and may delay early medical specialty referral to a neurologist to look for an underlying biological cause to the behaviors that may seem abnormal. In fact many children are not referred to a neurologist until three or four years of age. This may delay medical diagnosis and treatment options discussed in this book. Also current data support that diagnosis by rigid standards by age two is fairly predictive that the child will have autistic behaviors at age nine or later. Therefore, early intervention medically should not be delayed, and waiting for more time will probably not change the diagnosis.

The first step in describing a child with autistic behavior is to describe their nonverbal connection to their parents or caretakers. Children with early-onset autism may or may not be verbal. If verbal, many parents fail to recognize abnormal early language such as knowing the alphabet or saying "hippopota-mus" instead of saying "ma-ma." Often parents believe that such abnormal or "super-normal" language is a sign of intelligence. Children with early autism may never gesture, never reach out to be picked up, avoid hugging back, or require abnormally firm pressure when held. Some of my patients have even described their infants only wanting to be held as long as they face away from the parents instead of facing them. If present, waving or "peek-a-boo" games, pointing, flirting, or "patty-cake" games are very encouraging even in a child with delayed verbal expression of language, because these activities demon-strate shared social nonverbal language capabilities. Shared play interests evolve by 12 months of age, and this type of shared play is usually a good indicator of autism being less likely or of at least a milder degree of social impairment being present. Many parents who describe their children as regressing after 15 months, or who blame immunizations as a cause for autism, are never ques-tioned about the detailed nonverbal activities described briefly above. Careful attention to nonverbal communication history is important to document true regression.

Another significant error in diagnosing autism in very young children is the presence of global delays in gross motor skills as well as language. In the exten-sive clinical experience of my practice, children have often been referred to me with encephalopathic conditions such as cerebral palsy, brain malformations, myopathies, or other genetic disorders, whose parents believe their children have autism. Parents and primary care providers should not confuse global developmental delay in gait, motor, and speech development with autism. Sensory integration disorders are not unique to ASD, and children with cerebral palsy, seizure disorders, attention deficit disorders, Tourette's syndrome, and mental retardation all can have sensory integration disorders. Many conditions can coexist or cause autistic traits, and self-stimulatory behaviors such as hand flapping or rocking may exist in up to 5 percent of non-autistic children.

Parents often need the encouragement from pediatricians to ask about language and social development. It has been the recommendation of the practice guide set forth by the American Academy of Neurology and Child Neurology Society that parental concerns are usually accurate. By one year of age, any child not gesturing, babbling, maintaining eye contact, looking or responding to calling of their name, or having self-stimulatory movements such as hand flapping, is at risk for an autism spectrum disorder and should be referred to an appropriate diagnostic professional or center for autism. Only by using an appropriately trained physician can any underlying neurological diseases that overlap autism be ruled out. This cannot be accomplished by speech, occupational or physical therapists, psychologists, teachers, social workers, chiropractors, or other non-medical caregivers. In fact, in order to get insurers to pay for services in many regions of the United States, only a medical physician's diagnosis is recognized.

Parents and professionals should make their referrals as early as a suspicious clinical delay is noticed. There is no standardized universal method to confirm the diagnosis of an ASD, although psychological screening tools such as the Autistic Diagnostic Interview (ADI), or the Autistic Diagnostic Observation Schedule (ADOS) are usually quite predictive of the condition being present. These types of screening tests do not rule out other neurological conditions that may mimic autistic conditions. Therefore the simplest rule should be that if a parent is concerned, their child should be referred. For pediatricians in charge of infant care, at 12 months the question of language development, nonverbal gestures, play, and eye contact should be discussed with the parent at routine check-ups. To ensure that pediatricians or family physicians do this, every parent should be educated to ask about or confirm that language and social development is appropriate. Waiting to refer these children is, in my opinion, a factor in our lack of understanding what may cause autistic regression in the 12- to 18-month age group. If we knew every 12-month-old at risk, then those children that truly regress at a later age would be better defined. Parents who do not bring their child to see a child neurologist until three to five years of age are often not sure of the details of when autistic features manifested themselves. This has led to unfortunate guessing that maybe it was an immunization or some other factor such as diet, but none of this can, as of today, be retrospectively confirmed.

Case in point is that recently a physician I am familiar with, who himself has an autistic child, mentioned he knew a nurse with a child who immediately regressed after an MMR (measles, mumps, rubella) vaccination. I asked then why they hadn't been referred or self-sought help from a neurologist to look for a possible medical cause or confirm a possible immunization-related event. Because even this experienced professional did not raise the alarm and call for immediate help, this opportunity to intervene and evaluate for true regression and early medical intervention was lost. As a neurologist, I suspect this child may have had other causes, and the question of seizures or global encephalopathy from vaccine could have been established with early evaluation. This may be the "one in a million" immunization-linked encephalopathy, but not necessarily immunization-caused autism. It may also be a case of previously undiagnosed degenerative or a genetic disease such as Rett's syndrome or fragile X syndrome, or Batten's disease (see Appendix 2: Glossary for definitions). I encourage any pediatrician or family practitioner to refer with haste any child who regresses within three months or less of an immunization. Until this is done the medical community will not be able to answer with certainty the role of vaccinations in childhood autism. More on this topic will be discussed later, but I do not feel the evidence, as of 2007, shows that immunizations cause anything but a fraction of a percent of the current autism epidemic. In fact, if parents totally avoid immunizations, a measles epidemic will lead to thousands of deaths, and perhaps thousands more cases of post-measles encephalitis children with brain damage that may mimic autism, and polio and other vaccine-preventable diseases will come back. Whooping cough outbreaks are already occurring from this pattern of avoiding vaccinations in some areas of the United States, and a mumps outbreak occurred in 2006 in Iowa.

The diagnosis of autism is a clinical pattern of aberrant behaviors that deviate from normal social and language development. Currently the standard varies and can be made with or without expensive neuropsychological testing or observation. The predominant deficit for these children is in the realm of communication; understand that this is global loss, which is why gestures, sign language, or eye contact can be critical to differentiate a language-delayed child who cannot make speech from autistic delay. The inability to make speech is expressive aphasia, while the inability to understand speech is auditory agnosia or receptive aphasia. Partial impairment of these functions is when the term "dysphasia" is used. Complete loss of function to express spoken language with oral motor problems is "apraxia," while partial loss of motor speech skills is "verbal dyspraxia." Parents often are told their child has dyspraxic speech or apraxic speech based on the above, but sometimes dysphasia may be a better term. The majority of autistic children suffer from both receptive and expressive dysfunction. The most common complaint is when the child seems to act as if deaf to language. The child may be selective in hearing, such as when they hear television, but does not respond to spoken efforts to engage them. Often parents notice stereotypic behaviors such as hand or finger movements, toe walking, finger movement in front of the eyes, or spinning. Toy play may be restricted to carrying or throwing toys, lining or piling up toys, and not really playing in a typical way (such as holding or flapping a car but not rolling it on the ground imitating a real car). Aversion to eye contact, touch, or hugging, or to noises that are typical in daily living, may also be a significant observation.

Although these aberrant behaviors are often obvious, for first-time parents or parents in denial of their child's symptoms, the need to make them advocate for early evaluation by an autism diagnostic center or a knowledgeable child neurologist or child psychiatrist must be encouraged. The following sections will define further the standards of diagnosis and treatments. Remember there are no cures currently. However, with early diagnosis in the hands of capable child neurologists, child psychiatrists, developmental pediatricians, and even primary care physicians, there is the hope that medical diagnostic testing can be performed almost anywhere in the United States or any modern country elsewhere. The best scenario is the rare case where another treatable condition such as hearing loss or epilepsy is found and the child improves. Other conditions that may mimic autism may also be diagnosed, such as atypical attention deficit disorder, Tourette's syndrome, or severe childhood onset anxiety disorders, such as selective mutism. This book will further define simple steps for physicians to take to ensure a thorough neurological approach to that child being diagnosed accurately with autism. Remember that the key message for the rest of this book will center on the following facts: It is never too early to intervene, and appropriate medical evaluation is essential to maximize any other therapies that the child may need. If a parent or physician suspects autistic risk, even at the first birthday, sound the alarm and get help. I believe it is better to sound a false alarm than to regret waiting too long to start down the path of seeking appropriate medical care that each one of these children deserves.

PART II
Definitions, Diagnosis, and Other Clinical Aspects

Chapter 3

Defining the Clinical Aspects of Autistic Spectrum Disorders

In the prior chapter the clinical overview was given, but what standard techniques are used by schools, physicians, psychologists, and government agencies that diagnose or track autistic disorders? The focus of this chapter will be to discuss the different methodologies and familiarize the reader with these techniques. In no way does the clinical treatment or diagnosis require all, or even any particular one, of these screening tools. They are more critical, however, for future epidemiological work, or public sharing of information such as research to help define which subpopulation of autism responds to which type of treatment. These diagnostic tools do not differentiate between acquired or regressive autism, because they are only descriptive of the present level of function. None of these tools have been standardized to document changes in the degree of autism so they have limited value tracking treatment outcomes.

The first tool used universally and easily available is the *Diagnostic and Statistical Manual* of the American Psychiatric Association (DSM-IV) now in its fourth and latest revision. This is a guidebook representing the consensus of the American Psychiatric Association members that categorize neuropsychiatric disorders based on the criteria of having a specific number of symptoms that seem to define a disorder. This is based on clinical behaviors, not biomedical proof such as a blood test, brain neuroimaging, or genetic findings. Bipolar mood disorders, depression syndromes, attention deficit disorder, schizophrenia, and autistic disorders represent just a few of the conditions defined by these observational criteria. Down's syndrome would not be in this manual, even though dementia and retardation may exist, because there is a clear biological way to define that disorder. State agencies, such as California's Department of Developmental Services, use the DSM-IV to define autism in tracking the disease, and many research efforts in the past have used this as a standard to define disorders such as those in the manual. Clearly, the manual lists descriptive data, and does not prove useful to measure changes or cures of a particular disorder. If your child has been defined as having autism by this method, it only means that the child has enough of suspected behaviors to overlap with the DSM-IV definition. This does not rule out other potentially treatable conditions that may overlap with some of the various symptoms.

The criteria to diagnose autism from the DSM-IV require six items from three categories which describe behaviors seen in autism. The three major categories are:

1. socialization

2. impaired communication

3. repetitive/stereotypic behaviors.

The criteria for autism are also defined by onset at less than three years of age, but the DSM-IV does not differentiate regression vs. non-regressive subtypes. The latest version of the DSM-IV differentiates autistic spectrum disorders (ASD) (which it refers to as pervasive developmental disorders (PDD)) by autistic disorder, Asperger's syndrome, pervasive developmental disorder-not otherwise specified (PDD-NOS), childhood disintegrative disorder, and Rett's syndrome. Rett's syndrome, which is now defined by a biological genetic test, may be removed from future versions of the DSM manual.

The next major psychological tools used for diagnosis at major autism diagnostic centers are the Autism Diagnostic Observation Schedule (ADOS) and Autism Diagnostic Interview (ADI). These criteria were developed by psychologist Catherine Lord and her colleagues, formerly at the University of Chicago and now at the University of Michigan, in order to strictly define autism and differentiate it from PDD or other developmental delays. These are expensive and time-consuming, but are becoming necessary for ongoing research projects because they help standardize criteria for patients being treated for autism. These require special training, for the ADOS in particular, and further training for research application. These tools do not seem sensitive to mark changes in the disorder and are mainly defining the presence of autism. Again these are not necessary for clinical management of any autistic child, but are specific in defining autism as a condition. For many current and future researchers this testing is considered the "gold standard" to firmly unify research definitions of autism or ASD. When practical, as part of a diagnostic work-up for autism, this is a good baseline to obtain especially if your child may participate in an ongoing research trial. Clinically the diagnosis can still be made without this time-consuming testing. Remember, this testing must be administered by appropriately trained personnel in order to be considered valid. Despite the cumbersome nature of ADOS and ADI, recent follow-up shows they have good predictive ability for determining future risk and stability of the autism diagnosis from ages two to nine years.

The Childhood Autism Rating Scale (CARS) is a descriptive format questionnaire based on observations of the child's behaviors asked of the parent and has a statistical score which indicates the likelihood of autism. The Garland Autism Rating Scale (GARS) is again a questionnaire of symptoms but is broken up in three subcategories, including socialization and language/communication. These can be somewhat more useful in measuring changes in score over a three- to six-month period, enabling them to have some usefulness in research trials measuring change.

The main thing for parents to realize is that all of these diagnostic screening tools are confirmative and describe autism. These methods only describe the appearance clinically, not the underlying biology or cause. This is similar to describing someone's characteristics, such as: "How tall are they?", "What color is their hair?", and so forth. These questionnaires or diagnostic observations do not rule out other causes for these behaviors. There is still some subjectivity to all of these screening tests. These observational criteria do not take into account different medical causes for these behaviors; for example: infantile spasms, cerebral palsy, fragile X syndrome, infection of the brain (such as encephalitis), or mental retardation; and underlying medical conditions, such as intractable epilepsy or deafness, are not excluded or evaluated by these defining scales for autism. Yet all these medical conditions may overlap with the appearance of clinical autistic traits. If autistic traits are present but the child has a condition such as those mentioned, then they may meet criteria for an ASD, but this would be secondary to an underlying medical condition. These types of children are different from children presenting with autistic characteristics with no known underlying medical condition that has caused brain injury or dysfunction.

Asperger's syndrome, a variant of highly verbal high-functioning autism, can be diagnosed with the Australian Scale for Asperger's Syndrome, or the

Asperger Syndrome Diagnostic Scale, with both child and adult versions. These again are questionnaires with the score based on how the patient or caregiver answers the items. Biological causes or comorbid conditions such as bipolar disorder, attention deficit hyperactivity disorder (ADHD), obsessive disorders, anxiety, or depression are not excluded by these scales.

A good screening tool for one- to two-year-old children is the Checklist for Autism in Toddlers (CHAT), which is a brief questionnaire that only screens for possible autism. This is however a good tool for parents or pediatricians to think about if there are early signs by 12 to 15 months of age. Recently the Pervasive Developmental Disorder Screening Test for toddlers (PDDST) was modified for younger children with the PDDST-II. The PDDST-II was shown to be more predictive at 12 to 15 months than the CHAT for screening of autism at this young age. Therefore tools for early recognition are getting better and can be used even at the primary care level.

There are many other psychological tools this book and chapter will not detail. These explore motor, sensory, language, and intelligence measures such as intelligence quotient (IQ). These can be used at different ages for both verbal and nonverbal children to somewhat different degrees of accuracy. The final issue is the functional aspect of the child which may differ from these measured levels of capability clinically.

The overall usefulness of diagnostic screening tools for autism is that they offer statistical methods to confirm the likelihood of the diagnosis being correct. These scales do not really predict long-term outcome or treatment possibilities, or differentiate autism with regression from non-regressive cases nor do they separate primary from secondary autism based purely on behavioral measures. I refer to primary autism as having no other cause and this may include regressive or non-regressive type. Secondary autism has some underlying primary issue like cerebral injury or infection or genetic disorder that appears to have autistic behaviors clinically. For definition purposes in this book, autism with regression refers to children who start out for 15 to 24 months as having relatively normal social and language skills and then seem to lose these skills such as eye contact, language, or social abilities. The non-regressive type—the majority of autistic children—tend not to regress because their skills were always delayed or absent even in early infancy.

Chapter 4

What Type of Autistic Spectrum Disorder Does My Child Have?

The last chapter helped explain some of the diagnostic psychological criteria to diagnose someone with an autistic spectrum disorder (ASD). However, from a clinical point of view, there are ways to further subdivide the ASD subtypes. This is most important from a possible medical treatment perspective.

The clinical history and presentation of the individual child needs to be carefully documented by the parents and physician making a diagnosis of an ASD. From the point of view of differentiating these subtypes, there may be some clues in how the child presents with an ASD. Does the child start out with a normal pregnancy and delivery? Does the child have a history of medical problems as a neonate or infant? Did the child evolve normally from infancy during the first three to six months of life? How about six to twelve months of life? If completely normal at one year, then when did the child change to start losing social and communicative skills, and what other unusual or maladaptive behaviors did the child acquire?

Once the questions above are evaluated, a true clinical story of your child's experience relative to the world of ASD can be defined. For example: If your child had always been delayed in motor, feeding, social, oral motor, and language, then this is different from a child with normal motor development, but lack of eye contact and nonverbal social interaction only. Children who are completely normal in social and nonverbal infant skills through 12 to 18 months, who also acquire some proper language, then regress at 15 to 24 months of age represent still another clinical group of regressive type ASD.

These children are considered to make up about a third of autism cases, and are a group that requires a thorough neurological work-up when they regress. Again the idea of early intervention at the time of concern may allow better chances to medically treat and halt progression of this form of autism with regression. Remember, ASD is a spectrum disorder. One way clearly to keep this perspective in mind for me is a set of drawings of three children with different levels of autism that I have seen in my office. As seen in Figures 4.1, 4.2 and 4.3, these drawings represent the fine motor and visual motor ability of three autistic boys between 10 and 12 years of age. Given the variance in levels of ability and visual motor skill represented in this group, is it any wonder that diagnostic categories in ASD are broad, and that these labels represent a spectrum? Is it surprising that careful neurological evaluation may find different levels of motor tone, electro-encephalogram (EEG) differences, and different language ability among these children? Is it not intuitive that there would be no single treatment, but many different treatment choices medically to consider in this population? Table 4.1 summarizes the categories of ASD subtypes.

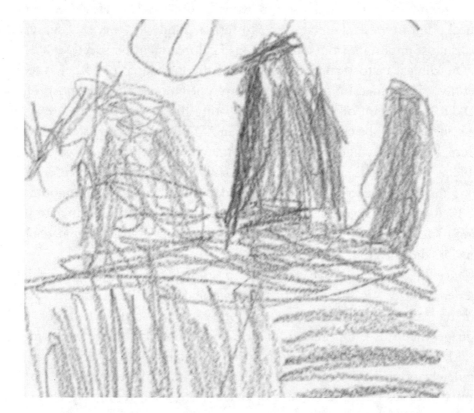

Figure 4.1: Drawing by a lower-functioning 10-year-old boy with nonverbal autism

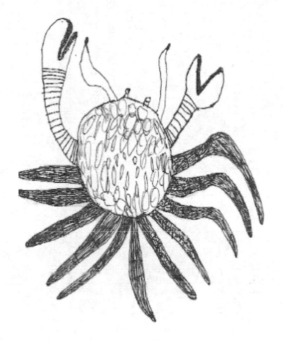

Figure 4.2: Drawing by a high-functioning 11-year-old boy with autism

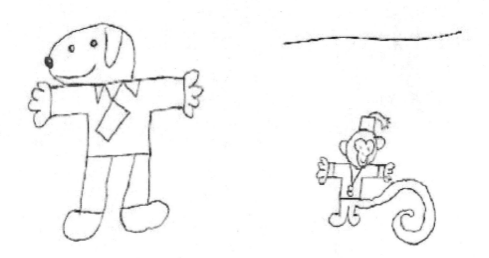

Figure 4.3: Drawing by a moderately impaired 12-year-old autistic boy with speech delay and mild mental retardation

Table 4.1 Autism subtypes

ASD subtypes	Non-regressive	Regressive	Asperger's	Secondary ASD
Age of onset	Birth to <12 months	>12 months, >18 months, >24 months	No regression, verbals often missed under age 2 years	Result of brain injury: asphyxia, infection, stroke, severe seizure disorder (infantile spasms), associated neurological disease (fragile X, Rett's, Angelman, for example)
Language deficit type	Expressive, Receptive Mixed Type or No Language Deficit	Loss of receptive often more than expressive, can be mixed type	Often fluent language	Can have oral motor apraxia, expressive language deficits more than receptive, although can have both or mixed types
Auto-immune role?	Not sure	+, suspected	– ?, not suspected currently	Not sure since multiple etiologies
When to evaluate?	By 12–15 months	As soon as aware of regressions	Usually at age 2–5 years	As soon as medical problems present
Abnormal EEG	±	+ Especially if >18 months of age when regress	Usually normal EEG	Often abnormal if epilepsy present

Non-regressive autism

This category is not really differentiated by the diagnostic evaluations that place a child in the ASD category. This is relevant in that early identification, even from newborn through three months, may indicate something is wrong. For example, these may be the quiet or "good" babies that never really cry or demand attention, or they can be the other extreme of constantly irritable or fussy. These children may develop some language but their nonverbal social skills are deficient. These children may know letters or numbers by 12 to 20 months of age, and some may even say names of objects. These children rarely attach to their parents or like being held; they lack reciprocal interests and may respond to music or a television show but have no interest in parents or family members. These children may show the desire for sameness. They often lack ability to play with a toy, but may carry a toy or object inappropriately. These children often start self-stimulatory behaviors after 12 months of age, but some may tense up their arms or hand flap between six months and one year.

These children may have a genetic predisposition for such an early onset, but they may also have suffered an intrauterine event, such as a stroke. At this time the reason for this type of presentation is unclear. In my own clinical experience, these children sometimes have abnormal sleep EEG patterns, but less so than in the regression group. Typical magnetic resonance imaging (MRI) and computerized axial tomography (CAT) scans are normal. These children almost always have normal gross motor development. Many of these children become verbal, but may have abnormal patterns of speech, including single-word utterances, echolalia, or rote phrases from book or video information. Some of these children may have savant skills or be hyperlexic (skills such as the math abilities in the movie *Rain Man* or reading before three years of age). In contrast, my clinical experience with the regressive subgroup does not have hyperlexia as a commonly seen feature. Often, in my experience, children with hyperlexia have more severe nonverbal social interactive deficits compared to the other subtypes as well. Gross motor milestones early on are normal, but these children may be clumsier later, have lower muscle tone, have difficulty with motor planning and fine motor skills.

Regressive autism syndromes

This clinical observation again is not differentiated by the classic autism diagnostic scales such as the Autistic Diagnostic Observation Schedule (ADOS) or Autistic Diagnostic Interview (ADI). This group may have some similarities to other degenerative neurological diseases. This group needs to have a thorough early neurological referral as close to the time of regression as possible. Various genetic and metabolic diseases may present in this manner. Metabolic disease may present with unusual need for excessive naps, fatigue, and excessively long sleep. Usually metabolic and genetic disease has motor delays as well as language regression or delay.

Differential diagnostic possibilities exist here. These include genetic conditions (e.g. Rett's syndrome, fragile X syndrome), degenerative diseases (e.g. mitochondrial or metabolic disorders including Batten's disease or adrenoleukodystrophy), epileptic conditions (e.g. acquired epileptic aphasia), encephalopathic seizure disorders (e.g. infantile spasms or Lennox-Gastaut syndrome), rare psychiatric conditions (e.g. child disintegrative disorder, early onset schizophrenia), also other conditions (e.g. lead poisoning, thyroid disorder, failure to thrive). These diseases are very rare as causes of ASD. Mitochondrial abnormalities (due to the energy producing parts of cells) may be 1–2 percent of autistic-like presentation, and some metabolic states are rarer, maybe 0.5 percent of cases seen. Therefore at the present time most cases will not have a definite cause. This is one reason that many fearful parents associate regressive ASD as possibly being associated with vaccinations or other common early childhood events.

For the majority of ASDs with regression in language, there is often a central auditory component with areas of the brain that process speech showing a clinical dysfunction in understanding spoken language. A common story typically seen in this group includes a loss of previously developing language. Often these children may not have had perfect language development, and they lag behind normal children to various degrees, including more receptive speech deficits or acting as if they become deaf. They may have fewer appropriate words, or make only word approximations or leave off syllables. In these cases it is critical to ask parents if they gestured or pointed in the past, and to what degree they were interactive at a social level before they lost communication or eye contact skills. Often there can be associated sleep disturbances at the time of regression or shortly thereafter. Sometimes these children may have been even older when they regress and a careful and detailed history of social skills and language can be critical. Differences in regressive and non-regressive ASD are shown in Table 4.2.

The critical factor in the regressive subtypes of ASD is to do a thorough medical evaluation and make sure there is no hearing loss, rule out exposure to lead paint, make sure you are not dealing with a genetic or degenerative

Table 4.2 Differentiating regressive from non-regressive ASD

ASD type	Age of onset	Language	Self-stimming	EEG abnormal
Non-regressive	<12 months	Delayed, atypical, or absent	Usually	Can be normal *or* abnormal
Regressive	>12 months	Normal or abnormal then lost		Can be normal *or* abnormal

disorder, and make sure no epilepsy is present if clinically suspected. This group was once thought to be much more likely to have an abnormal EEG, especially if the regressive behaviors begin after age 18 to 24 months. More recently, more detailed and larger studies using 24-hour EEG recordings have not been able to differentiate the rate of EEG abnormalities to be higher in autistic children who regress over 18 months of age versus those who do not regress. There still may be higher rates in regression over 24 months of age, but this is a much smaller subgroup. More will be discussed on this later. In addition, this group may be associated with the latest theories of chronic or acquired activation of an inflammatory response in the brain, which may in theory lead to this regression. I believe this group may be very well studied in the next few years with markers for inflammation in the blood or spinal fluid. More on the possible mechanism of regression is discussed in Chapter 12 on immunology and autism.

Asperger's subtype

This subtype is often not diagnosed until later preschool, or even up to junior high school age in some cases. Language is often fluent and the child may seem even pseudo-mature and very knowledgeable at an early age about topics such as dinosaurs, trains, motor vehicles, or other areas of narrow interest. These children are sometimes delayed in speech initially as well. They have little interest in socializing unless it relates to a topic of interest. This group has normal to above average intelligence quotient (IQ) scores, but the idea of these children being above average or genius level is a myth. This group may have trouble with spelling and phonics, but not be bothered by background noises. This may differ from high-functioning autistics, where there is good phonetics, but problems with background noise discrimination. Self-stimulatory behavior can be present in both Asperger's and high-functioning autism. High-functioning autism usually has more language delay and is usually diagnosed earlier in life. Asperger's patients do not have a history of regression. There is no biological test to identify this group genetically or physiologically. Epilepsy is rare in this group, and EEG findings are typically normal in Asperger's patients. Asperger's patients may also differ in response to medications.

Secondary ASD

This subtype is becoming more discovered as medical and genetic advances are being achieved. The old categories of Rett's, fragile X, and Angelman syndromes are now genetic entities. Other medical groups such as Smith-Lemli-Opitz syndrome, Lesch-Nyhan syndrome, Williams syndrome, and other conditions are now diagnosable as genetic conditions (see Glossary to define these diseases). This differs from the 1970s when often these disorders would be included in the clinical phenotype of ASD. Another rare group of metabolic disorders now identifiable by medical spinal fluid testing includes children with motor regression, seizures and autistic features. These may be part of now diagnosable neurotransmitter disorders, and more recently folinic acid deficiency. These are rare and only diagnosable by spinal fluid. Identification is important when clinical features are present with motor regression and sometimes seizures, especially because these conditions are at least partially treatable.

Landau-Kleffner syndrome (LKS) is a rare form of epilepsy where nocturnal EEG is disturbed and clinical seizures may occur, and children lose their language. This medical condition is seen in older children (ages three to six years) without earlier onset of autistic features. Other forms of epilepsy are now known to affect language and development, and seizures beginning in infancy, such as infantile spasms with or without the comorbid condition of tuberous sclerosis, can be highly associated with mental retardation and also autistic development. Lennox-Gastaut type epilepsy can also be highly associated with autistic characteristics. These epileptic groups differ from idiopathic autism in that there is early onset of frequent and often severe epilepsy, and the EEG can have rather severe features of epileptic patterns not seen in children with ASD only. Epileptologists are frequently reporting the presence of poor social and language development in children with early-onset seizures, especially if before age two years. Many medical articles now describe how epileptic activity can disrupt learning and behaviors, both from actual seizures and from the presence of epileptiform activity on EEG tracings, in between or in the absence of clinical seizures.

Early-onset global delay as seen in cerebral palsy or in brain trauma or asphyxia is also a possible reason for erroneous labeling of children as having an ASD. In these cases there is clearly an organic brain lesion or injury involved. Neuroimaging may reveal lesions to the brain or developmental evidence of brain ischemia or malformation. The clue to this type of pattern is when there is both global motor and language delay. Most true idiopathic cases of autism do not also have significant gross motor delay. Many globally delayed children have more oral motor involvement, yet receptive language may be present as well as social ability nonverbally. This pattern may also help differentiate this group from early-onset autism.

Some genetic disorders may also have autism secondarily. These include Down's syndrome, Rett's syndrome, Angelman syndrome, Praeder-Willi syndrome, fragile X syndrome, Smith-Lemli-Opitz syndrome, and Sotos syndrome among others. These are all identifiable by genetic testing clinically available. These are not primarily autism, but have autism characteristics as part of their syndrome.

Summarizing the important facts of this chapter is that ASD comprises different degrees of impairment, and one third may regress at a later age over 15–24 months of age. Newer genetic tests may help remove certain diseases that have autistic characteristics from the ASD categories. Knowing that motor delays are not typical of classic autism may also be a clue to look for underlying medical brain injuries, metabolic, or genetic disorders.

Chapter 5

Current Recommendations
for Medical Evaluation

As a practicing pediatric neurologist who specialized in epilepsy, I started evaluating autistic children who happened to have either seizures, late regression and abnormal electroencephalogram (EEG) findings, or children with language regression resembling Landau-Kleffner syndrome (LKS), a rare medical condition with language regression usually between ages three and five years. More will be discussed on this later. When I began to evaluate children with autism as recently as 1990, there were no guidelines for physicians such as child neurologists or child psychiatrists to follow. Starting in 1998, three guidelines have been produced with differences reflecting the bias of the groups recommending the medical protocols.

The first group to tackle the daunting task of a standard medical approach stemmed from a meeting sponsored by the charitable foundation Cure Autism Now (CAN). This was published in 1998 and set forth the following recommendations. Primary care providers should screen 12 to 18-month-old children with tools such as the Checklist for Autism in Toddlers (CHAT). In cases with receptive speech delay a hearing or audiological evaluation should then follow. Lead screening was recommended even though this is very rare. Again all of the above do not require a specialist such as a neurologist. Recommendations then follow to refer to an autism specialist, either an accredited child neurologist, child psychiatrist, developmental pediatrician, or a medical center based developmental program specializing in autism. A thorough medical history, birth history, family history, and medical and neurological exam should be performed on each child suspected with autism. No specific genetic screening is recommended by the CAN Consensus Group unless clinical suspicion for fragile X or other genetic diseases is evident. Neuroimaging, such as computerized axial tomography (CAT) scan or magnetic resonance imaging (MRI), was not recommended as routine unless the neurological exam or EEG turns out to be abnormal. Also CAN's expert panel recommended at least an EEG with six to eight hours of sleep to determine fully if any EEG abnormality that may be contributing to language deficit or delay is present. This is recommended for any child delayed or regressive in speech, or suspected of clinical or subclinical seizures. Various metabolic testing, such as amino acids, urine organic acids, thyroid functions, lactic acid levels, carnitine levels, and any other suspected tests for allergies, etc., is at the discretion of the evaluating specialist. The CAN group does not recommend a "shotgun" approach and asks specialists to use clinical judgment in metabolic or genetic testing.

Also in 1998–1999, the American Academy of Child and Adolescent Psychiatry established their own guidelines. These guidelines are very biased for early screening, suggest a lead test globally, but do not take as aggressive a stance regarding genetic, metabolic, neuroimaging, or EEG screening as do the other groups. Reflecting a lack of their experience in EEG in clinical practice, the child psychiatry group recommends an EEG only if clinical seizures are present. Hearing evaluation was also recommended.

The most authoritative medical recommendations so far subsequently have come from the American Academy of Neurology and Child Neurology Society (AAN/CNS) with a group consensus guideline published in 2000. These guidelines again recommend early screening at 12 to 18 months, audiologic evaluation, and early use of the CHAT, the Autism Screening Questionnaire for children four years of age or older, and the Australian Scale for Asperger's Syndrome for high-functioning children who may have gone undiagnosed. Other screening tools are currently being evaluated, but are still being validated. Diagnostically, this consensus statement has similarities to the CAN Consensus with regard to testing. Neuroimaging is recommended only with clinical suspicion of a neurologic deficit or EEG abnormality; lead screening where suspected; fragile X and chromosomal karyotyping in all patients; and metabolic screening similar to the CAN statement. EEG testing is recommended with samples of stage 2 and slow-wave sleep in children suspected of developmental regression or suspected seizures.

As you can see, these medical guides leave room to vary the work-up for patients individually. None of the medical group guidelines recommend specific treatments or even when to treat with medicine. For instance, even with a neurologically abnormal EEG in sleep, there is still no agreement when to treat with an anti-epileptic drug in the absence of clinical seizures. Again, we hope that the subsequent discussions will help delineate treatment options.

The medical community does not feel there is any substantial evidence linking mercury poisoning from thimerosal in vaccines to autistic spectrum disorders (ASD). In fact, the type of mercury in thimerosal may not even be biologically available for absorption. In addition, there has never been any evidence of mercury poisoning in any child that I have seen in 15 years of practice who received chelation therapy from alternative practitioners. Therefore screening for mercury and heavy metal intoxication is not recommended.

There is no true evidence that gluten, wheat, or milk sensitivities cause ASD. None of these factors have made a difference in my experience in medically treating ASD. In fact even in biopsy or laboratory-proven celiac disease cases that I have seen with ASD, no symptomatic improvement has occurred to the autism features from the gluten- and casein-free diet. Certainly, if parents elect to try this course of treatment they should discuss taking celiac blood tests and RAST (radioallergosorbent test) allergy testing for wheat, gluten, and dairy before undertaking such a restrictive diet. Because of a lack of any clinical evidence of causation in ASD from these dietary issues, no consensus group of scientific medical origin has current recommendations to test for these allergies in the absence of strong clinical or family history of these conditions. There is no reason to test for yeast or metabolites of yeast as a cause of autism either from a scientific basis.

Therefore, my recommendation is to use the CAN and AAN/CNS guidelines as a template and vary individual factors when discussing your child with a specialist. Adding a pervasive developmental disorder screening test-II (PDDST-II) is reasonable for 12- to 18-month-olds as well as the CHAT. My bias is definitely to do the overnight or six- to eight-hour sleep EEG as it may offer a treatable subtype within autism, or at least qualitatively improve receptive speech and sleep when certain types of nocturnal EEG abnormalities are present. These will be discussed in a later chapter. These tests are easy to perform, so there is no reason to deny any parent access to a quality EEG given today's digital technology. Do not take no for an answer on this test. I do not believe there is any medical credence to the tests being offered by alternative medical practitioners who claim to have tests for treating autism, such as tests for mercury poisoning or so-called chemical imbalances that have not been discussed by the mainstream medical community as having validity. If in doubt, check with groups like Autism Speaks, the American Academy of Pediatrics, the Child Neurology Society, American Academy of Neurology, or American Academy of Child and Adolescent Psychiatry as resources if you have doubts about the research or medical advice being given. Also the National Institutes of Health in the United States offers information. Many universities with autism diagnostic centers may also offer information on these topics. I feel these types of internet or public sources have the best resources without commercial or unproven bias for potential help for parents and professionals wanting more information about autism and medical options.

Chapter 6

The Role of Medical Laboratory Diagnostic Testing

The diagnosis of your child having an autistic spectrum disorder (ASD) is an observational clinical diagnosis. At this time there is no specific diagnostic chemical, genetic, brain imaging, electroencephalogram (EEG), blood, urine, or tissue sample that confirms a diagnosis of autism or differentiates autism from other developmental disorders. That being the case, there is a useful way to use laboratory, neurophysiological, and radiology testing to rule out other conditions that may mimic ASD. This chapter will focus on laboratory testing.

Laboratory testing includes blood and serum (fluid in blood without the blood cells), genetic, urine, and spinal fluid samples that give medical information. The sections that follow are a guide to some testing that may be routinely ordered by a doctor when evaluating autism. Summaries for which tests are essential to be done and which tests are optional or situational will be outlined. The laboratory tests most useful in the current medical evaluation of ASD are shown in Table 6.1.

Hematology

Hematology is the study of blood for diagnosis of blood disorders. The usual test is the complete blood count (CBC). The CBC reflects bone marrow function and nutrition, general health, inflammation, or underlying disease by the values of the types of blood cell formation. Simple blood tests for hematology or analysis of the patient's general blood health is important at baseline, since medications that can change blood cell values may be used in the treatment of ASD. In addition, clues about the child's general health will be obtained. This helps to rule out anemia, and other blood disorders. It also may give clues to nutrition or other genetic diseases, vitamin deficiencies, or other problems, such as blood loss from a gastrointestinal or kidney problem. Infection or inflammation can also be crudely assessed. Hemoglobin and hematocrit, and red blood cell morphology help assess anemia, iron deficiency, and bone marrow activity. White blood cells assess infection fighting ability, bone marrow function, and whether exposure to viruses or chronic inflammatory states is present. Platelets are blood clotting cells that may be abnormally high with autoimmune states or low due to some medications or bleeding disorders. Also with medications the bone marrow may sometimes be affected, so monitoring is a good idea for safety. Because of the importance of these medical indications a CBC should be checked in all patients presenting with ASD behaviors.

Metabolic blood chemistry testing

Basic blood chemistry, called routine metabolic testing in most hospitals, is usually also ordered by your physician as part of the general work-up. A comprehensive metabolic panel normally includes information on body sodium, potassium, chloride, urea, and glucose balances. It also gives information on protein nutrition, kidney and liver function, and acid-base balance. Sometimes, mildly low bicarbonate levels may represent an underlying state of increased acidosis in the body. This is sometimes associated with underlying metabolic diseases like mitochondrial defects or organic acidemias. Rarely, mildly elevated liver function tests may represent mitochondrial dysfunction or toxin exposure or liver infection. Most of the time mild elevations or decreases in these values mean nothing. Some tests may include bone or calcium information. Special tests may be added for cholesterol levels, iron levels, or other mineral levels. Some rare diseases, such as Smith-Lemli-Opitz syndrome, may have low cholesterol levels and autistic features. Some poorly sleeping autistic children or children with restless legs syndrome may have low iron levels.

Other tests, referred to as metabolic screening tests, include those for lactic acid or pyruvic acid levels looking for rare conditions such as mitochondrial disorders. Mitochondria are energy-producing sites within your body's cells; they are metabolically important to brain, liver, and muscle tissues, and how they function. Amino acid levels can be obtained in order to rule out rare protein

Table 6.1 Practical laboratory tests in ASD

	Hematology	Serum chemistry	Genetic	Immunology	Urine	CSF
Commonly performed tests	CBC, differential	Electrolytes, glucose, thyroid functions, lactic acid, carnitine level, amino acids	More often where suspected: Fragile X (boys); high resolution karyotype; Rett's (girls)	In cases of frequent infection: Immunoglobulin levels; TNF-alpha; sed. rate	Organic acids	Regression with neurotransmitter or degenerative profile
Additional tests secondary to clinical findings		Zinc copper, iron, possibly when suspect	Rarely when suspected: Angelman, tuberous sclerosis, other diseases. Future: microarray?	T-cell subtypes; anti-nuclear antibodies (ANA); cytokines		Future may become routine?

metabolic disorders. Phenylketonuria (PKU) is screened in newborns and is one example of a metabolic disorder that may present as an ASD. Blood sampling may be requested by your physician to look for vitamin deficiencies, such as vitamin E, A, B12, folic acid, or others. Screening for blood levels of metals such as zinc, copper, iron, or lead may be ordered in specific cases by some physicians where deficiencies or toxic exposures are suspected. Serum levels of lead may give a clue in children where risks of lead ingestion are historically a risk because of living in a house with paint containing lead and a history of pica. Pica is a condition of eating unusual things like dirt, paper, aluminum foil, sand, or other non-edible substances. Sometimes zinc, copper, or iron deficiency can be seen with pica. Zinc is rarely low, but a deficiency results in rashes and developmental delay. Some vitamin deficiencies cause types of dementia. Those include deficiencies in vitamin B12, folic acid, vitamin E, vitamin A, phytanic acid, and other nutritional factors that may be screened. Carnitine deficiency can yield low tone in muscles or low energy, and also may reflect an underlying metabolic deficiency or a possible mitochondrial disease. Although sometimes these are found to be abnormal in some individual patients, no specific patterns exist in autism.

Blood tests for hormonal function

Hormonal disorders most associated with developmental delay include thyroid disorders. Screening may include testing thyroid stimulating hormone (TSH) that is produced in the brain pituitary gland, T4 or T3 levels or uptake to check the thyroid gland itself, and thyroid specific antibodies where autoimmune thyroid disorder may be present in the family. Diseases that are very rare such as Addison's disease, or adrenal leukodystrophy, may present with developmental problems and cortisol deficiency. Some parathyroid hormone levels may be abnormal with developmental delays in children. Also rare insulin-producing tumors may cause low blood sugars, which may mimic seizures or delay development or cognition. Abnormal parathyroid hormone levels have been associated with retardation and seizures. Most of these conditions rarely overlap the autism diagnosis. However, most neurologists will usually screen the thyroid functions as part of a comprehensive evaluation. This is even more important if there is a maternal history of an autoimmune thyroid condition such as Hashimoto's thyroiditis. This condition of thyroid deficiency has been associated in some families with autism.

Immunological functional testing

The immune system is now becoming more suspect as a site of potential influence on brain development and also as a possible mechanism in causing autistic regression. Unfortunately, there are few good blood tests to help because peripheral blood may not reflect the central nervous system cells and immune system that is regulated by the neuroglial, not peripheral immune cells such as T- and B-cells from the blood. Only by extrapolating indirect evidence can we make theoretical connections in certain clinical types of ASD where there may be forms of systemic low immune response and frequent clinical infections.

Simple blood tests for immunity include getting a CBC. This test gives basic levels of white blood cell number and types. Eosinophils are elevated in allergic conditions, and elevated types of other white cells crudely reflect bacterial versus viral type exposure. An erythrocyte sedimentation rate (sed. rate) reflects nonspecific inflammation, as does a C Reactive Protein level about the general state of inflammatory response in the body. T-cell subtyping reflects the total number and function of pro-inflammatory type lymphocytes vs. inflammation-inhibiting types of cells. B-cell counts reflect types of cells that make antibodies that fight diseases or inflammation. It may be useful to measure any natural killer cells in the blood to look for activation of these inflammatory cells. Total immunoglobulin levels and levels of IgG subtypes may reflect global immune susceptibility to infection. Elevated IgE may reflect allergic or parasitic problems. These tests should be case selective and are certainly not for all children with autism, only when there are specific immune questions like recurrent infections, failure to thrive, chronic diarrhea, and other conditions that may warrant questioning a child's immune function.

The products of activated inflammation, including cytokines, are just beginning to be understood, and some of these tests are being developed for clinical use in autism in research laboratories currently. Proteins called antibodies may reflect specific or nonspecific levels of reaction against the body itself or infection. Many doctors look for celiac disease or gluten sensitivity by ordering anti-gliadin antibodies. With anti-gliadin IgG elevated in nonspecific ways, it does not mean a patient has wheat or gluten sensitivity unless the anti-gliadin IgA type of antibody is also elevated as in celiac disease. A more sensitive tissue trans-glutamase test is more accurate in the diagnosis of celiac-like conditions. This has been an area of confusion for many parents, in my experience, and often makes people interpret that wheat/gluten sensitivity is present. The elevation of IgG gliadin antibodies is nonspecific and may represent some cross-reaction with other autoimmune reagents occurring within the patient. Myelin basic protein or anti-neuronal antibodies are sometimes elevated in the blood of some patients with ASD, but spinal levels of myelin basic protein are negative in ASD; therefore this is yet another example of the peripheral blood immune system differing from the immune system seen in the central nervous system. Serum antibodies against capillary nuclear cells have been described in research blood tests but are not commercially available. Some of these antibodies also react with Brain-Derived Neurotrophic Factor (BDNF), but this is not yet commonly commercially available at hospital laboratories. Anti-nuclear antibodies (ANA) are elevated in the disease called lupus, and rarely elevated in ASD. Tumor Necrosis Factor alpha (TNF-α) in the serum is being evaluated but does not clearly have meaning at the present time. BDNF and TNF-α may have important roles in brain glial cells and neuronal migration and development. In a small case series of 12 autistic patients, cerebrospinal fluid levels of TNF-α may be elevated, but the meaning is unclear at this time. Certain animal models also implicate these cytokines in the development of epileptic neuronal activity. Abnormal elevated levels of BDNF have been found in cord blood samples in ASD children in one research study. Despite future promise of these types of immune tests offering guidance in ASD treatment, at the moment these factors are only being studied in research laboratories. These are not currently recommended tests for ASD.

Currently, preliminary data on only a limited number of spinal fluid studies have been published, and even fewer brain tissue samples for inflammation have been studied. However, and especially in cases of ASD with regression, there may be elevated cerebrospinal fluid levels of inflammatory proteins such as certain cytokines like interleukins IL1, IL2, IL6, TNF-α, BDNF, and macrophage chemoattractant protein (MCP-1). The future holds much potential for improved research into immune mechanisms involved with ASD. Spinal fluid testing may soon become a standard rather than the rare sampling that has been done in the past.

Genetic testing

The excitement and heavy investment in human genetics has yielded the completion of the human genome project, genetic therapies, and improved understanding of many previously identified diseases or their risk factors. Genetically inherited diseases like Huntington's disease, Duchenne muscular dystrophy, and many neurodegenerative diseases have been found to show specific genetic markers, which can be tested for using commercially available laboratory tests. Unfortunately there are no tests for specific single genetic markers commercially available for autism. At the present time at least 22 chromosomes are identified for ASD. Previous conditions such as fragile X, Rett's syndrome, tuberous sclerosis, Angelman syndrome, Prader-Willi syndrome, Williams syndrome, and other types of diseases with ASD overlap have been identified by genetic markers or tests, and these are commercially available. However, these may represent only 1 to 5 percent of cases identified as ASD. The rest of the types of ASD remain unidentified with at least 22 suspected genetic links or markers, including small deletions on chromosomes 2, 6, 7, 15, and 22 and the X-chromosome among others. This may explain why genetic testing is suggested mainly to rule out suspected cases resembling fragile X, Rett's, or Angelman's. For most patients with ASD, these tests are negative in the absence of clinical features. Despite recent availability of genetic tests, no male Rett's cases have yet been identified and this remains a disease that affects only females. These tests help only to eliminate these specific disease types from other ASDs that currently have no specific genetic testing available. Just recently new clinical microchip genetic array analysis screening panels looking at multiple telomeric genetic deletions are now possible, and hundreds of genes and the full chromosomal karyotype can be studied by a single blood test. These newer tests may reveal more information in previously negative genetically tested patients with dysmorphic appearance and ASD. Most recent consensus is that these new techniques show maybe 10 to 15 percent of children with an ASD may have some spontaneous microdeletion genetically, but these are not yet identifiable as causative for autism. More is discussed in Chapter 9 in this book. Most current consensus groups limit recommendations to run genetic karyotypes or fragile X testing in suspected cases. If Rett's syndrome is suspected, then this should be run. For most doctors, genetics remains a secondary testing as in most cases the yield has been small in clinical application up until recently.

Body tissues

At the current time it is only recommended to get skin or rectal tissue biopsies in degenerative cases like Batten's disease (ceroid lipofuchinosis), or sometimes in cases with suspected lactic acidosis or mitochondrial disease. Muscle biopsy is recommended in suspected cases of mitochondrial disease only. There is no role for brain biopsy at this time in ASD diagnosis.

Gastrointestinal biopsies via endoscopic upper or lower gastrointestinal studies are recommended to rule out diseases where severe intestinal diarrhea, or severe constipation are noted. This would help rule out celiac disease, eosinophilic gastroenteritis, and other types of inflammatory colitis. It also helps rule out gastroesophageal reflux and ulcers common in this population. Again these gastroenterology tests must be clinically warranted.

Urine tests

The most common urine tests in ASD would be the quantitative urine organic acid test. These and other tests can show suspected lactic acidosis and other very rare metabolic disorders. For most cases of ASD these tests are normal. Tests of urine for yeast metabolites or gluten and casein sensitivities are not recognized by traditional medicine as having any value. There are currently no FDA-approved tests for urine to test for mercury poisoning unless severe acute toxicity within 24 hours of exposure. Those tests that are being used for screening have not been shown to be useful for chronic or past exposure to mercury. Therefore, unless the patient was just exposed acutely to mercury poisoning, the meaning of these tests may be inaccurate. Chelation-induced urinary tests for excreted toxic materials have not been standardized for normal children and have no real scientific merit in ASD. Collecting urine for heavy metal toxicity for 24 hours can be done in most hospital laboratories, but again there are no proven cases of mercury or metal toxicity in the medical literature associated with current or prior cases of ASD despite the media hype. In one fairly large series of collecting urine from autism cases and controls looking at environmental factors at the MIND Institute, no differences in serum or urinary mercury levels have been found so far between autism cases and controls.

Cerebrospinal fluid studies

Until recently, performing lumbar puncture for evaluation in ASD was rare. In the absence of suspected metabolic or degenerative rare diseases, this has not been done. In the past few years some cases of neurodegenerative patterns with movement disorders, seizures, and PDD have gotten cerebrospinal fluid (CSF) studies looking for types of neurotransmitter disorders. There have been a handful of cases with cerebral palsy type of motor development, autistic features, and sometimes seizures found to be deficient in folinic acid in the CSF. There have not been any studies of CSF in large numbers of ASD children, but past literature and modern experience suggest that common markers for elevated CSF cell counts, immunoglobulin, myelin basic protein, oligoclonal bands, protein and glucose levels are usually normal. Specific levels of transmitters such as glutamate levels or other neurotransmitter metabolites have not been well studied. Pre- and post-treatment effects of medications used to treat symptoms of ASD have not been studied by looking at CSF either. Future testing may include routine CSF studies looking for cytokine subtypes, and evidence of neuroglial activation of autoimmune type. This is not currently being recommended, however. In cases of suspected neurotransmitter deficiency or folinic acid deficiency, a spinal fluid study is the only way to make the diagnosis.

Hair analysis

There are no controlled studies of any type to support the validity or usefulness of hair analysis in diagnosing or treating cases within the ASD spectrum. In a controlled adult study, hair specimens sent to three different commercial laboratories showed no correlation even with the same samples. In my almost 20 years of clinical practice, I have yet to see a consistent or convincing clinical pattern from alternative hair analysis laboratories that showed any clear evidence of lead or mercury poisoning in my autistic patients. No published research based on hair analysis and its use in treating autism exists currently.

Allergy testing

In cases of suspected food allergies or in cases of eosinophilic gastroenteritis, careful skin and serum allergy testing is needed. There is little evidence that assays of multiple food IgG sensitivity screening are valid or meaningful for ASD treatment. Having an abnormal IgG sensitivity is not the same as a true food allergy, such as seen in an IgE-type food allergy. People with many IgG sensitivities are not necessarily allergic to those foods. Many chiropractors and alternative therapists are using these meaningless tests to design diets or add supplements. There are no known thermocoupled or light-fluorescent allergy tests that are valid by just holding a light device. When allergies are suspected, a thorough allergy evaluation by a competent pediatrician or board-certified allergist is recommended.

Stool analysis

In the presence of chronic diarrhea or gastrointestinal bleeding or similar distress, stool testing is best used for determining the presence of parasites or pathogens in standard hospital laboratories for ruling out infection. There has been no standard agreement among traditional pediatric medical practitioners or gastroenterologists for defining whether there exists true yeast infection or dysbiosis or abnormal overgrowth, despite the claims of several popular alternative laboratories that provide nearly the same ASD diagnosis to everyone who sends a sample. Anaerobic bacteria require special sampling techniques not commonly performed at any commercial laboratory. There is no evidence that yeast or bacteria commonly found in stool samples sent by mail for analysis cause ASD. These overgrowths may reflect the techniques of collection and mailing the samples, allowing yeast and certain bacteria to overgrow.

Chapter 7

Neuroanatomy
and Neuroimaging

What is neuroanatomy and neuroimaging?

Neuroanatomy refers to the shape and structure of the central nervous system. In autistic spectrum disorder (ASD) there has been no unified agreement about a specific neuroanatomic deficit or error in development that by gross appearance of the brain would correlate to having ASD. The structures that have been studied consist of the balance center or cerebellum, the brainstem, the frontal lobe, the temporal lobe (especially the mesial area that interacts with memory and emotion), and the limbic connections. Microscopic anatomy or pathology has been studied in a little over 30 brains from a national autism brain tissue depository. Only qualified researchers have access to this material. The initial studies that were published described brainstem cell tract losses, cerebellar Purkinje cell loss, mesial temporal lobe cellular changes, and disrupted frontal lobe tracts. There was no description of inflammation until recent studies on ten brains showing neuroglial inflammatory changes. No specific white matter changes were described. These earlier findings conclude that perhaps intrauterine insult occurred at about 27 weeks' gestation during fetal development, but newer imaging and pathology studies do not necessarily agree with this theory. In fact, recent immune data suggest that Purkinje cell loss may be a result of neuroinflammation. The initial neuroimaging focused therefore on the cerebellum and other areas described above. More recent neuroimaging has focused on functional changes in the higher cortex and grey or white matter structure.

Neuroimaging refers to describing tests available to measure brain morphology, metabolism, biochemical, or functional modalities. There are clinically applicable brain image or morphology scanning techniques that are available at most medical centers in the United States and developed countries. Most of the specialized brain imaging research that is published for ASD theories is undertaken in academic research facilities, with access only to patients participating in a particular research study. This limits what the typical ASD patient has access to get done at the current time within their communities. Often the research published in the media or scientific journals describing brain morphology changes in size, white matter, or metabolic activity is done in specialized research centers where it remains unavailable to treating physicians. This occurs even at clinics for ASD within the same university medical centers where the specialized neuroimaging often takes place. This chapter will focus on both areas of neuroimaging: The tests available in the community, and tests used in research.

Community-based neuroimaging tests

Neuroimaging consists of brain morphology studies, most commonly to analyze for gross defects in brain development or structural integrity. In the past these were computerized axial tomography (CAT) scans and rarely skull x-rays. Magnetic resonance imaging (MRI) is now the standard way to view brain anatomy. This gives better views of the white matter (the myelin or insulated fiber tracts that carry information from brain cells) and the grey matter (nerve cells regions of the brain). MRI also gives better views of posterior brain regions thought to be involved in autism, such as the cerebellum and brainstem, than CAT scans could in the past. These scans are good to rule out hemorrhage, stroke, and developmental structural defects, but do not show activity of brain function in routine MRI studies.

MRI spectroscopy (MRS) is a newer way to image chemical spectrums within areas of brain and can look at the brain chemistry of many neurotransmitters or their byproducts. Newer higher Tessla-powered magnets for MRI machines will allow greater biochemical studies using MRS in the future, due to their potentially greater resolution capabilities. This may allow doctors to compare pre- and post-treatment MRS patterns of certain chemicals such as GABA, glutamate, or creatine that may be monitored. In addition, differentiating white matter inflammatory processes may be identified with MRI diffusion technology techniques.

Functional MRI (fMRI) is the technique of doing an MRI in a cooperative patient while doing a cognitive or simple motor task. Obviously this technique can only currently be applied to cooperative patients and therefore limits the usefulness to high-functioning patients with ASD or Asperger's patients. Currently this technique is helping to define areas of speech, motor function, reading, memory, and attention in the brain.

Positron emission tomography (PET) scans of the brain map functional areas based on glucose utilization rates or other chemical markers that measure metabolism or receptor differences in different areas of the brain. This can also help determine function by, for instance, different metabolic rates in different areas of the brain while doing a task. Currently the PET scan does not seem to yield major usefulness to guide treatment, but visualization of gross changes in the brain functionally that may be altered by pharmacotherapy to some degree can be imaged. This allows PET scans to follow levels of certain brain receptors to dopamine or serotonin, for example. Clinical use of PET has mainly been limited to research purposes so far.

Brain nuclear spectroscopy (SPECT) measures radioisotope blood flow activity in different parts of the brain. In certain types of central nervous system dysfunction due to autoimmune vasculitis or encephalitis, decreased SPECT regional blood flow may reflect underlying small blood vessel inflammation. An example of this is in the condition known as Hashimoto's thyroiditis with encephalitis that shows inflamed areas with decreased microvascular blood flow changes. CNS lupus also can show this type of change. SPECT scans are an older technique and are more widely available at smaller hospitals. Clinical routine MRI and CAT scans are also now widely available. Less commonly available are fMRI, MRS, or PET scans. Another technique that can measure epileptic potentials and function is brain magnetic encephalography (MEG). This type of scan may be very useful in the future, but is still very rare outside of research applications, and has probably been underutilized in ASD. One study compared Landau-Kleffner electroencephalogram (EEG) localization to the interictal spikes seen in ASD with regression. This type of data is very rare overall.

In practical terms, current guidelines have not found significant abnormalities in standard MRI or CAT scan findings in most cases of ASD. Unlike research findings where certain cerebellar structures are smaller for example, or certain white matter tracts are enlarged, the usual community neuroimaging results do not find this to be the case. PET and SPECT, MEG, and fMRI or MRS are not currently recommended or necessary for the diagnosis of ASD. However, research to understand better ASD etiology and subtypes in certain research centers has been making progress using these more advanced techniques. The bottom line is that in most cases, without bedside evidence or neurological or EEG abnormalities, the MRI is usually normal in most clinically studied cases of autism in the community.

Neuroimaging research studies and results

Past research started in earnest with CAT scan availability. This documented larger brain size and smaller cerebellar vermis (midline structure) in earlier studies. Currently the gold standard has been MRI scanning with comparison to normal volumetric averages to support differences between ASD and control populations. MRI studies have focused on the cerebellum, brainstem, total brain and frontal lobe volume, temporal lobes, and, more recently, asymmetries and grey–white matter differences.

The cerebellum was initially focused upon because of theories of retrograde brainstem damage and repetitive behaviors seen clinically in ASD. The cerebellum is a primitive brain structure involved in balance and coordination, as well as primitive learning. Lesions to the cerebellum in animal models and in human patients have revealed the cerebellum may be involved in certain behaviors seen in ASD, as well as in rudimentary language-learning processes. Limited brain tissue pathology studies have shown decreased numbers of Purkinje cells and granular cells in the cerebellar cortex. This has been the incentive to study the cerebellum with neuroimaging. Some studies have suggested that the vermis (middle cerebellar structure) is smaller compared to normal non-ASD controls. While some studies have shown this, other researchers have had difficulty reproducing these findings. Other studies have even shown some enlargement of the cerebellar lobes that surround the vermis. Despite the inconsistent reporting on different studies, the overall consensus in the research literature is that the cerebellum shows some degree of vermal volume loss. This finding may support other theories in ASD regarding autoimmune, ischemic, or neuroregulatory defects since the Purkinje-type cells are more susceptible to these types of injury or dysregulation.

More recent studies have looked at the connection from the cerebellum to the frontal cerebral cortex. These studies have shown increased frontal lobe volume with decreased cerebellar size. The exact relationship of these observations is not yet clear, but many explanations may exist. Some scientists hypothesize that the frontal lobes grow to compensate from a lack of input from the cerebellum. Other explanations may be that an immune process injures the cerebellar Purkinje cells causing volume loss, while frontal white matter increases volume to compensate for neuronal loss in the grey matter. These theories are still being explored and questioned.

MRI brain growth/volumetric studies

Even in the early descriptions of autism, enlarged head circumferences were observed. One study found that 90 percent of autistic boys aged two to four years had a head circumference greater than 95 percent of controls. However, at least one recent study has not found head sizes to be different between autistic and control patients. Some recent MRI studies have shown that there is indeed increased brain volume. There is also evidence that the observed increase in brain volume may in fact be due to abnormal increased white matter, particularly in the radial white matter that borders the grey neuronal areas. This is especially true in the inferior frontal regions. There is also an observation of the reversal of volume in the frontal language areas in language-impaired autistic patients compared to controls with normal language development. Normal subjects have more white matter volume in the left frontal lobe; while language-impaired patients with ASD have shown greater volume in the right frontal regions. This is a reversal of normal asymmetry. Other non-ASD language-impaired patients also showed this trait. This suggests early language disruption leads to an effort by the brain to compensate in the mirror region of the opposite hemisphere.

Other studies of brain growth in ASD have been done. These show earlier white matter and brain volume growth increase up to two years of age in ASD, while in non-ASD controls growth is present later at ages two to four years and nine to twelve years. This may explain early increased head sizes seen in ASD that are not present in adulthood relative to normal controls. Also it shows a deceleration of white matter and other growth after an abnormal early start. This suggests a possible disrupted neuroregulatory mechanism in ASD subtypes, although the exact mechanism is still unclear. Intrahemispheric U-fibers are more affected than interhemispheric connections. This increased deep white matter is thought to be compensatory, not necessarily making deficits better, reflecting dysfunction of the overlying grey matter. A schematic drawing of these regions is shown in Figure 7.1.

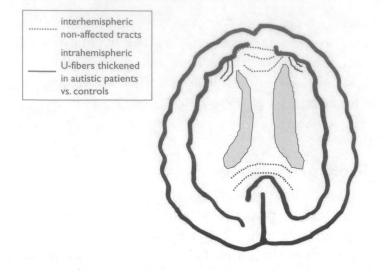

interhemispheric
non-affected tracts

intrahemispheric
U-fibers thickened
in autistic patients
vs. controls

Figure 7.1: Brain white matter tracts

Brain organization in functional neuroimaging

PET scan and fMRI studies have shown disconnection between frontal lobe areas and asymmetric activation of tasks such as language. Suggestions that areas of the brain activate in isolation almost as islands of activity without the normal interconnections have also been made. The left inferior lateral cortex is the location for Broca's expressive speech area. The lateral posterior temporal lobe and planum temporale are sites of Wernicke's receptive speech area. The deeper opercular area in between these sites is the location of oral motor function for producing speech (see Figure 7.2). These areas are clearly shown at risk in MRI, PET, and fMRI studies showing reversed asymmetry, or decreased activation of these language areas. Early loss of receptive speech activation has been studied using PET scanning in children from orphanages where early sensory and language neglect led to decreased activity over Wernicke's area functionally. Many of these children suffered from "institutional autism", or acquired behaviors associated with this early environmental language depriva-tion that led to autistic behaviors. More theories on the possible susceptibility of these areas to injury will be discussed in other chapters.

Studies using fMRI in higher-functioning young adults with ASD demon-strate decreased activation in the left frontal and parietal cortex for complex memory tasks compared to normal controls. Complex sentence tasks show

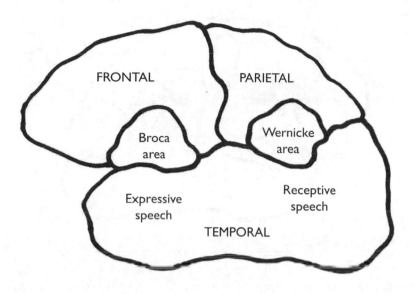

Figure 7.2: Schematic drawing of major speech areas in the left hemisphere

fMRI decreased activation changes again to the left frontal cortex and increased activation in an abnormal fashion over the receptive speech regions in the left hemisphere (Figure 7.3). These changes are a reflection of disorganized regions that because of some injury or misdirected neuronal circuitry have inefficient auditory processing and subsequently less recruitment of activation of the expressive speech regions. Similarly, supplementary motor planning activation has also been abnormal in ASD patients using similar fMRI techniques when compared to controls. Recently, fMRI studies at the University of California at Los Angeles (UCLA) have shown abnormal activation of the area of the operculum called the pars reticularis, which is the location of the "mirror neurons" that allow imitation of emotional facial expression to occur. This site does not show normal activation in autistic subjects compared to normal controls. This suggests abnormal development of this important area that connects facial motor function to the limbic emotional response centers in the brain. This area is near the expressive speech area connections and a region important to oral motor skills called the insular cortex.

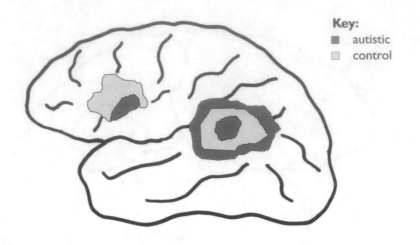

Figure 7.3: Schematic drawing of regions of increased receptive speech area activation and decreased frontal expressive speech activation as representative of known fMRI patterns seen in ASD young adults

Biochemical patterns found in neuroimaging

Biochemical markers have been searched for utilizing PET and MRS. Some MRS research has focused on creatine transferase deficiency in non-ASD language-delayed patients. This has not been found in ASD, however. Epilepsy studies have shown decreased GABA levels, and elevated homocarnosine levels, but this has not been studied yet in ASD. PET scans have shown dysfunctional patterns of metabolism, and also abnormal serotonin metabolism in younger children with ASD. These PET studies have documented increased serotonin metabolism in younger ASD patients, with slowed rates of serotonin metabolism in adolescence and adults. No clinically useful interventions have so far resulted from these studies for patients with ASD. Future higher-powered MRI magnets and better computer technology will hopefully allow better biochemical studies utilizing MRS. Some early studies show abnormally high glutamine and lower glutamate conversion. Some higher Tessla-powered magnets also show abnormal creatine levels, though lower-powered MRI magnets do not show this pattern typically.

Magnetoencephalography scan studies

Magnetoencephalography (MEG) scanning is a relatively rare technique that utilizes magnetic imaging and the electrical fields that record electrical activity from the brain similarly to EEG; in essence it combines some of what MRI and EEG tests each do. MEG has rarely been employed to date in ASD. It has been gaining popularity in pre-surgical epilepsy and in certain areas of neuropsychological research. One study showed that in non-ASD children with language dysfunction and abnormal EEG findings, the left temporal region near Wernicke's area showed localization of epileptic spikes. In another study, children with ASD and abnormal EEG patterns with sleep-activated epileptic spikes on EEG were compared to children diagnosed with Landau-Kleffner syndrome (LKS). The localization of the ASD children's spikes was similar to the LKS group. This did not conclude these were the same disease, only similar localization. Functional testing in ASD with MEG has not been utilized to date, but may offer future research potential.

Neuroimaging conclusions

Practical use of neuroimaging at this time is to use MRI to rule out gross anatomical structural abnormalities in patients with ASD and focal neurological deficits or abnormal EEG findings. Most clinical guidelines currently do not recommend routine neuroimaging in ASD. There are no recommendations for routine use of fMRI, MRS, PET, SPECT, or other tests, such as MEG scans, at this time. Quantitative white matter volume measurements are not widely available for clinical purposes. The research findings described are not currently clinically available, nor at this time do they affect treatment decisions for symptoms of ASD. It is hoped that future research will help understanding of the cause and possible treatment of ASD. Future neuroimaging technology then may be clinically warranted in the diagnosis or treatment phases for patients with ASD.

Chapter 8

Electroencephalography

The Relationship of Epilepsy or Epileptic Activity

The relationship between epilepsy, abnormal electroencephalogram (EEG) patterns, and autism dates back to initial observations by Dr. Leo Kanner in the 1940s. Through the subsequent years many authors have reported medical observations of increased rates of abnormal EEG in higher percentages of ASD patients than corresponding normal population experiences. As patients with autism grow up to adulthood, up to one third may experience clinical epilepsy (consisting of at least two or more seizures clinically). Early neurological descriptions of the relationship between autism and seizures, and the presence of abnormal brain wave patterns on EEG, called attention to the fact that autism is an organic brain disorder, and not just a psychodynamic or environmental deprivation disorder. However, even today, the exact role of EEG abnormalities and epilepsy in this population is poorly understood, not uniformly studied, and treated randomly; and long-term outcome is not understood to differentiate subpopulations of ASD with and without epileptic activity. It is well established that children or adults with lower intelligence quotient (IQ) scores, and/or with more profound neurological deficits, may be more impaired and may have an increased risk for physical epilepsy.

This chapter will try to explain what EEG testing can and cannot tell us about autistic spectrum disorders (ASD). I hope that the myths of this test being traumatic or impossible to perform on children with ASD will be dispelled. This diagnostic test is probably the most frequent abnormal test that can potentially be performed in patients with ASD. This chapter will argue that EEG testing should probably be part of every ASD patient's medical assessment.

Frequency of EEG abnormalities or epilepsy in ASD

Prior to the 1990s, the majority of EEG data came from large population data collections from Scandinavia or Australia utilizing short one- to two-hour EEG studies. Sleep EEG data was often missing. Sometimes studies were only analyzed in populations of ASD that had suffered an epileptic attack. Even with these limits, the historic facts were that ASD populations had a 30 to 60 percent chance of having abnormal brain waves or epileptiform activity on their EEG studies, and a 10 to 30 percent chance of having clinical epilepsy as they aged, specifically by adolescence or adulthood. For purposes of this and subsequent discussion of EEG abnormalities in ASD, I am referring to specific patterns on EEG recording that resemble spikes or spike-wave phenomena seen in epileptic disorders. The EEG patterns discussed in this chapter have similar morphology to known epileptic patterns or epileptiform activity. Figure 8.1 shows some different examples of this epileptiform activity from patients studied with ASD. Since the early 1990s, there were breakthroughs in technology allowing more accurate digital recording with hospital-based or ambulatory EEG for prolonged periods up to 24 to 72 hours. This was often done in early childhood or in cases of ASD that showed a clinical regression. The logic for this idea was an awareness of a rare condition that caused language regression in the presence of nocturnal EEG abnormalities and sometimes clinical seizures. This was Landau-Kleffner syndrome (LKS), which was first described in 1957. Unlike autism, LKS presents after three to six years of age with prior normal social and language development, followed by a clinical loss of language and sometimes what appears to be an acquired functional deafness or loss of receptive language. Classically it is associated with a specific sleep-activated EEG pattern of continuous abnormal spike-wave discharges in 85 percent of stage 2 and stage 3 sleep. This condition remains truly rare and is part of a spectrum of language and psychiatric disturbing EEG/epilepsy syndromes known as disorders of continuous spike-wave in sleep syndromes (CSWS). No autistic patients in my clinical experience have had this late-onset disease or pattern that classically fits LKS or CSWS conditions.

With improved prolonged EEG and clinical monitoring being more readily available since the late 1980s, reports began to emerge showing epilepsy rates between 5 and 30 percent in ASD, and peak times in early childhood, but also at early adolescence to early twenties. There was also observation that with prolonged EEG, especially capturing at least six to twelve hours of sleep, more epileptiform activity was found even in the absence of clinical seizures. Figures 8.1 and 8.2 show examples of the types of nocturnal sleep epileptiform activity found in ASD. In fact, the frequency from various centers performing prolonged EEG in this population shows a 40 to 60 percent rate of sleep EEG being abnormal in children with ASD, especially in subgroups that regress over age 18 to 24 months. In patient populations where clinical epilepsy has occurred, the frequency of epileptiform activity on prolonged EEG has been consistently greater than 60 percent, even with brief EEG recordings. I have recently published data on 889 ASD children without prior seizures or known medications and no prior abnormal EEG in the clinical history. The group averaged four years in age at their initial overnight EEG testing, and there were abnormal EEG patterns in sleep in 60.7 percent of the initial EEG studies. This is the largest collection of prospective EEG data to date in a low risk, young, prospective ASD

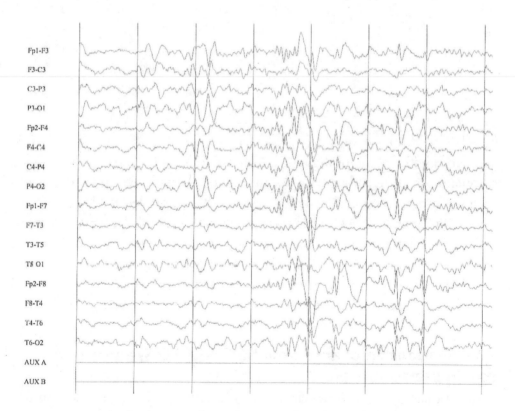

Figure 8.1: Example of right temporal central and secondarily generalized spike-wave discharges in an ASD patient

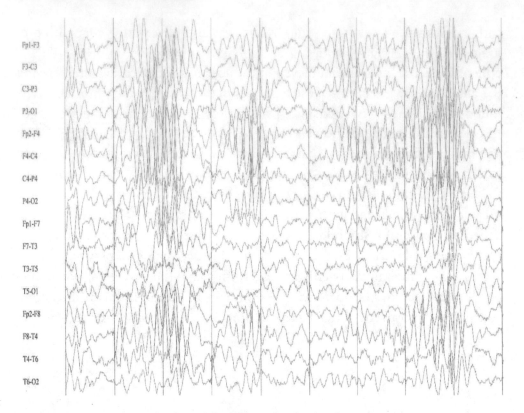

Figure 8.2: An ASD patient with secondarily generalized polyspike-wave activity

population without prior epilepsy risk factors clinically. This study is the largest case series with overnight digital EEG reported to date. There was no definite correlation to differentiate between the age of parental reports of regression versus non-regression in this study. These observations reflect the high percentage of EEG abnormalities seen in this population even in the absence of clinical epilepsy, and reflect that ASD has a definite organic brain dysfunction as a core component physiologically. The exact effect or clinical need to treat these abnormal EEG epileptiform patterns in sleep, in the apparent absence of clinical seizures, remains a topic of debate.

The relationship of abnormal EEG to ASD symptoms and role in regression

As mentioned above, the similarities for regression and language loss in one third of autism cases, and the high incidence of abnormal sleep EEG, has raised the question whether some subgroups of ASD resemble, or are in fact variant forms of, LKS. There are profound differences in these populations, with LKS being very rare, definitely less than 1:10,000, while ASD may be 1:100 to 1:200 births. In addition, LKS occurs after language is acquired, the epileptic patterns appear at later ages (age three to six years), and regression in language occurs in the absence of other features of autistic behavior. LKS has a 60 to 70 percent incidence of associated clinical seizures, while early childhood ASD cases with abnormal EEG patterns may have 10 percent presentation with clinical seizures. The frequency of sleep-activated EEG spike-wave abnormalities are defined as 60 to 80 percent of sleep being affected in LKS, while the frequency in ASD is rarely close to that, and the classic CSWS pattern used to strictly define LKS has never been described as present in ASD. Despite this, one study using magnetoencephalography (MEG) data showed localization to the posterior temporal and planum temporale areas for children with regressive ASD and sleep-activated spikes. This is the same localization as seen in LKS with both MEG and surgical descriptions. Some epileptologists believe the spike-wave phenomena of CSWS and the spikes in ASD patients are only epiphenomena. This means that the epileptic activity is reflective of some underlying problem in the brain, perhaps inflammatory or other causes. These doctors believe that the epileptic patterns on EEG are not directly related to the behaviors seen in the condition. Some authors have made the observation that ASD patients who regress have a higher incidence of abnormal EEG in the absence of clinical seizures than ASD patients who do not regress—19 percent vs. 10 percent respectively in one study. This was statistically significant. However, no data were offered on whether treatment was given and whether this would have led to different outcomes vs. ASD patients with normal EEG findings. At least two studies do note more EEG similarities to LKS when age of regression is factored into the patient history. Older regression after 18 to 24 months more closely resembles a variant of LKS. However, two recently published reports have found similar rates of EEG abnormality in both groups with regression after 18 months of age, and also in those ASD patients without observed regression. Therefore the rate of EEG abnormality may not depend on age of regression.

The summary of this data essentially shows that EEG epileptiform abnormalities are present in high percentages averaging around 20 percent with routine sleep short duration EEG and 50 to 60 percent of prolonged sleep EEG in preschool-aged samples with and without regression. These abnormal EEG patterns are usually seen in sleeping not awake portions of the EEG in ASD. The incidence of EEG abnormalities is higher if clinical epilepsy has been present.

The types of abnormalities most often seen are temporal-parietal or temporal central spike-wave abnormalities, or frontal sharp waves. More rarely seen are frontal generalized epileptiform discharges.

There is very new research in ASD looking at the role of certain inflammatory factors, including cytokine proteins such as interleukins, tumor necrosis factor, and Brain-Derived Neurotrophic Factor (BDNF). These proteins have also been described in cerebrospinal fluid, cord blood, and brain tissues of ASD patients. These and other similar proteins, and abnormal regulation of glutamate and N-methyl-D-aspartate (NMDA) receptors, have been described in animal models of epilepsy, as well as ASD. This may suggest that the epileptiform activity seen in some ASD subtypes may be a reflection of an inflammatory process that can disrupt brain function and affect neuroplasticity, cellular interconnections, neuroregulation, and potentially cause the promotion of epileptic-type activity. These recent research findings, coupled with the profound amount of EEG data, may be a clue to the linkage between the ways the brain is damaged in some types of ASD, and how the epileptiform EEG patterns may reflect further exacerbation of that process theoretically. More research looking at these similar mechanisms of inflammation in epileptic conditions and ASD should and will be done in the near future.

The main take-home message is that a prolonged EEG is probably important to obtain in any child regressing or presenting with a receptive language delay and ASD. In my clinical experience, the Asperger's population with more fluent language and later diagnosis tends to have infrequent EEG abnormalities compared to other ASD subtypes. More aggressive requests for prolonged ambulatory EEG should be done by physicians and parents advocating for children with ASD. The excuse that these children cannot tolerate such testing is a myth. In my practice 200 to 300 tests per year of ambulatory 24 to 48 hour EEGs have been performed since 1994. There is no reason not to obtain an EEG in any child with ASD on the ground they will not cooperate. When obtaining a prolonged EEG, sedation is not needed for sleep, so no medication artifact from sedation is present that may alter the EEG abnormalities.

EEG correlation to neuroimaging studies

The finding of abnormal EEG in the ASD population almost never has a structural abnormality of the brain morphology on magnetic resonance imaging (MRI) scans obtained after the EEG is performed. This suggests that EEG patterns seen are not simply due to obvious anatomical damage as seen after stroke or infection, or from brain cell malformation (dysplasia) from neuronal migrational abnormality. Therefore, abnormal EEG activity in ASD is a bio-chemical or microscopic abnormality of affected neuronal interconnections in the cerebral cortex. In a series of brain nuclear spectroscopy (SPECT) scans looking at cerebral cortical blood flow, I found decreased blood flow correlating to areas of spike activity found on EEG 83 percent of the time. This may be a reflection of microvascular or capillary inflammation in that area, but that is speculative.

MEG scanning of children with language regression and abnormal EEG found multifocal areas of disturbance correlating to EEG localization in 75 percent of the patients studied. Brain PET studies have not been well docu-mented to correlate to specific patients with abnormal EEG. In a small series of MRI spectroscopy (MRS) patients with abnormal temporal EEG spikes, there were no changes in chemical spectral arrays as seen in temporal lobe epilepsy in a small series of language-impaired children with ASD. Therefore, in most cases routine MRI is normal despite the EEG having abnormalities in these subtypes of ASD.

Conclusion

The presence of EEG abnormalities is more frequent in sleep than previously thought in the ASD population. The correlation to sites of social or language dysfunction, particularly brain areas related to speech reception or production, such as the centrotemporal regions, is potentially of clinical importance. Func-tional SPECT, functional MRI (fMRI), and MEG findings may also correlate to areas of EEG dysfunction. Although not yet conclusive, a history of regression is not necessary as a risk factor to have an abnormal EEG. The EEG spikes may represent cerebral dysfunction and perhaps another layer of immune-derived damage to the brain in autism similar to inflammatory mechanisms that create spikes in the epilepsy research currently being studied in animal models of epilepsy. Whether treatment of these EEG abnormalities alters the risk for seizures through the lifespan or changes cognitive or language in ASD patients has yet to be conclusively proven clinically. Treatment issues will be discussed later in this book.

Chapter 9

Genetics

The area of greatest research investment in autistic spectrum disorder (ASD) since the late 1990s has been in genetics. The human genome contains 22 chromosomes from each parent plus the sex chromosomes (X, Y) for a total of 46 chromosomes. Currently there are no single clinically available genetic tests or genetic markers linked to specific types of ASD. In fact, currently genetic markers are limited to small familial subgroups or other conditions with ASD features such as fragile X, tuberous sclerosis, Angelman syndrome, Rett's syndrome, and a few others. Most cases of autism and pervasive developmental disorder (PDD) have normal chromosome testing at the current time using commercially available laboratory screening tools. There are at least 22 chromosomal sites being studied in ASD. These will be discussed below. It is unlikely genetic therapy is going to be available in the short-term future. This chapter is almost like reading a new foreign language as genetic terminology is developing so quickly. For lay readers, I suggest you just use this chapter as a reference, and for professionals use this as an overview of what we can summarize about autism genetic research as of 2007.

Inheritance of ASD

ASD is one of the most inheritable conditions based on twin and family studies. Monozygotic or identical twins have a 90 percent correlation for inheritance if autism occurs, while non-identical twins have 10 percent correlation. The risk within families for a recurrence of a subsequent ASD child is 2 to 6 percent. This however may be artificially lower than actual figures because some families may stop having more children after having an affected child so there are fewer actual chances for a recurrence. The *phenotype* of ASD is how the patient looks and acts clinically, yet there may be different genetic causes for a single phenotype. The genetic pattern is the patient's *genotype*. There is also a broader phenotype which is a clinical spectrum of some ASD features that may run in family members to a less significant clinical degree. This can include other psychiatric conditions, like anxiety, social phobia, perhaps obsessive-compulsive traits, and mood disorders.

Unlike some disorders, ASD is a spectrum. This makes a simple single gene/single disorder unlikely. Also the phenotypes seen clinically are heterogeneous, not all the same. The genetic study of ASD has therefore included conditions that have ASD features, but are separate genetic and clinical conditions.

Other diseases with known genetic markers and ASD features

Scientists have studied known genetic diseases with some ASD clinical features, and have discovered the former DSM-IV pervasive developmental disorder, Rett's syndrome, has a genetic identifier on the X-chromosome called MECP1 region. This area has also been described in some non-Rett's patients with autism or retardation as well. This knowledge has helped move this previously confusing disorder into a new diagnosable and testable category separate from the global ASD group. Fragile X syndrome is similar as a cause of male retardation with some autistic features. This should decrease the rate of ASD being diagnosed, but as it is now known, despite better genetic knowledge to remove previously lumped conditions from the ASD pool, the rate of ASD has still risen to 1:166 births. The conditions previously included in the ASD category that are now separate entities include fragile X syndrome, tuberous sclerosis, Rett's syndrome, Angelman syndrome, Williams syndrome, and other disorders, including Sotos and Smith-Lemli-Opitz syndromes. Very recently identified genetic disorders include PTEN gene disorders and ARX genetic disorders that have associated mental retardation, seizures and often autistic behaviors. Older storage conditions such as the mucopolysaccharide disorders have also been separated from current idiopathic autism.

Fragile X is limited mostly to males and may overlap 2 percent of ASD cases diagnosed. The incidence is 1:3500 and clinically presents with more motor hypotonia and hyperactivity associated with the delay. There can be abnormal frontal epileptiform activity on electroencephalogram (EEG) that differs in localization from the EEG findings in the majority of typical ASD. Girls are mainly carriers but rarely affected. Cases are almost always male, therefore, because of the X-linked condition. X-linked diseases affect males more often because males only have a single X-chromosome, while females get an X from both the mother and father so a normal X-chromosome may override the abnormal X. In my practical clinical experience and those of my colleagues, I may have actually found fragile X only twice in almost 2000 cases of ASD screened genetically. Both times these were clinically suspected by maternal inheritance history or clinical presentation as atypical autism in a male.

Tuberous sclerosis (TS) is a condition with variable clinical phenotypes and can present with seizures, characteristic skin lesions, and brain tumors (benign tumors) that are often causes of epileptic activity. When presenting with infantile spasm seizures, this condition has a 90 percent mental retardation rate and a high incidence of ASD features. Mental retardation and partial seizures in TS are also associated with some features of ASD. However, some patients have well-controlled or no seizures, normal mental function, and no ASD features. The TSC1 and TSC2 genes are located on chromosome 16. These genes are on the short and long arm of chromosome 16 respectively, and may be involved in neurogenesis or migration. Some weak links to some autism cases have been found for the TSC2 region, but this is not conclusive and needs more verification. In other recent genetic studies, chromosome 16 has been linked in a small percentage of autism cases.

Rett's syndrome is a condition limited to girls and linked to the X-chromosome. This is the MECP2 gene site, but it has also been seen in some males with X-linked retardation, and 2 percent of non-Rett's phenotypical girls with ASD. The clinical phenotype of Rett's syndrome is a normal start developmentally, followed by an arrest of head and brain growth, and usually seizure onset and regression by age two years through four years. Lifespan has been usually only into the 20- to 30-year range in the past. Perhaps 30 to 40 percent may not have the arrest in head growth or stereotypical hand or breathing patterns seen in classic Rett's syndrome. This is exceptional as an X-linked disease, since the males with the marker are so rare clinically, probably because this defect must be highly lethal in male fetal development because males have only a single X-chromosome.

Angelman syndrome is a condition also called "Happy Puppet Syndrome" because of stereotypic facial and dental appearance. These children are mentally retarded, have seizures, and are usually friendly socially, with more global delay and hypotonic motor function than seen in ASD. This is usually associated with a severely abnormal EEG with generalized or multifocal polyspike-wave patterns on EEG, clinical seizures, and mental retardation. A defect in the neurotransmitter gamma-aminobutyric acid (GABA) is suspected. This is linked to deletions in the chromosome 15q region, and overlaps an area also causing Prader-Willi syndrome. Prader-Willi syndrome is usually associated with hypotonia and motor delay as an infant, light or blond hair, mental delay, and sometimes features of pervasive developmental disorders (PDD). As these children get older they begin to compulsively eat and get obese. These diseases are separate from rarely found ASD cases with 15q duplications. These cases are usually maternally derived and have been described in some families where there are autistic features, facial dysmorphic features, possible seizures, and often hypotonia. The incidence of 15q duplication is again rare and probably 1 percent of ASD.

Other genetic syndromes that can mimic ASD are hypomelanosis of Ito, Sotos syndrome (large head, mental retardation), Williams syndrome (elfin appearance, often aortic heart defect, chromosome 7, small stature, usually friendly), Smith-Lemli-Opitz syndrome (low cholesterol, unusual faces, mental retardation), and some metabolic disorders such as PKU (phenylketonuria) or SSADH (succinic semialdehyde dehydrogenase deficiency), a GABA defect that seems to cause mental retardation often with seizures.

ASD genetic links

Genetic research has generated over 500 scientific articles related to ASD since the 1990s. A major focus of the fundraising of the charity Cure Autism Now has been the formation of the Autism Genetic Research Exchange (AGRE). This with government cooperation has led to major new research breakthroughs, especially in getting large numbers of families with more than one affected child to donate and make available genetic material for research. This has led to genetic linkage studies of multiplex families that look for susceptibility genes for ASD. There are at least 15 to 20 of these genes that have been identified, and perhaps many more smaller genetic variants that lead to the broader familial phenotypes.

Techniques for genetic research have included whole gene scanning looking for a common site to turn up; investigating suspected genes with biochemical reason to be suspect in some symptoms of ASD; and looking for endophenotype analysis where a specific trait, such as language delay or obsessive traits, are focused upon within familial subgroups.

The whole genome linkage has consistently found some linkage to chromosome 7q. Other suspect gene sites include chromosome 2q, 4, 13, and 17p by this method. Candidate genes have been GABA (gamma-aminobutyric acid, an inhibitory amino acid neurotransmitter) receptor genes on 15q (GABRB3); SCL25A12 (on 2q, code mitochondrial glutamate and aspartate carrier); HOXA1 and HOXB1 (possible brainstem formation and abnormal dysmorphic appearance); SCL6A4 (17q, serotonin transporter gene SERT); RELN (7q, reelin protein involved in cell and synaptic migration/formation) and some other lesser reproducible links based on certain families. Language delay has been associated with chromosomes 2q, 7q, and 13q. Insistence on sameness has been associated with chromosome 15q GABRB3. Obsessive-compulsive traits are associated with chromosome 17 serotonin genes (SERT).

Recent findings of two additional genes have also shown that if you have one of these genes you may have perhaps double the risk of having an autistic child. One of these genes interacts with the immune system; the other affects chromosomal repair mechanisms. Again these recent findings are not clinically being screened in the general public at this time. The researchers admit that these genes need to interact with unknown environmental factors as well. These recent findings warrant watching.

Although the terminology is confusing and hard to understand, the take-home message for the reader is not memorizing the gene sequence terms or names. Just recognize patterns that affect different clinical behaviors associated with different genetic sites, and try to realize how complex these genetic variations can be even within families. At the current time, there is no single genetic link that is always present in a patient diagnosed with autism.

Clinical tests

The tests that physicians can commercially order now include a standard chromosomal analysis or karyotype, and fragile X testing for males. Rett's genetic testing for females, especially where clinically meeting the criteria, is easily available. Tests for Angelman, Williams, Sotos, Prader-Willi, Smith-Lemli-Opitz, tuberous sclerosis, and other rare conditions are now available. Advances in testing over the last three years means commercial testing with easy to obtain genetic arrays for sub-telomeric deletions and multiple genetic defects as well as karyotypes is available, allowing hundreds of deletions or genetic defects to be tested for on a single blood test. Recent evidence in some medical centers suggests that up to 15 percent of children with ASD have been found to have spontaneous new microdeletions by this method. Although the meaning of these various findings is still unclear, it raises the question of whether this type of testing should be done on every child with ASD. Clearly if unusual appearance or clinical history suggest a possible genetic problem, then these types of test may reveal new findings previously unknown in the ASD population. Only more clinical experience with this new technology in the field will see how useful these tests will become diagnostically.

Genetic conclusions

The most important take-home message about the current clinical state of genetics is that there are tests to diagnose other conditions that mimic or overlap ASD, but no commercially available tests to see if your child has a specific marker for ASD. With over 20 candidate genes and multiple variables, it is not going to be a simple puzzle to find a single unifying gene that places someone at risk for ASD. The genetic clues may help produce clinical subgroups that can guide certain therapies, like better response to one type of drug than another. This is still not available. Certainly all of these genes may be influenced to degree of dysfunction by environmental factors that are not yet fully understood. The research on the human genome and the overlap with autism genetic linkages will surely lead to more knowledge in the future about the complex spectrum of disorders we refer to as ASD.

PART III

Theories on Autistic Spectrum Disorders

Chapter 10

Why Are Autistic Spectrum Disorders Increasing?

The incidence of autistic spectrum disorders (ASD) is estimated to be somewhere between 1:100 to 1:200 births currently in the United States. Almost every state has shown an increase since the early 1990s. California state records show over a 600 percent increase through 1999, and subsequently another rise of almost that much again through 2004. Illinois went from 52 cases per year to over 5000 per year in the same period. Many claim almost every other state has had similar increases. Data from the Individuals with Disabilities Education Act had statistics showing an 871 percent increase in the incidence over the decade 1992 to 2002 for affected children from six to 21 years of age. There are some who try to pass this off as better diagnostic ability, and this may be partially true. Recent publications argue that there may be a diagnostic substitution with mental retardation and learning disabilities going down over the same time except in a few states. One of the reasons for this is that the Autism Diagnostic Observation Schedule (ADOS) and Autism Diagnostic Interview (ADI) are screening tools that are very inclusive and may take milder cases with other neurological conditions, such as tuberous sclerosis for example, and include such a child as also having autism or pervasive developmental disorders (PDD). From my clinical perspective, I believe these tests and screening tools do over-diagnose autism as the primary problem if you do not place another diagnosis, such as a chromosomal disorder, cerebral palsy, or chronic severe seizure disorder, as the primary diagnosis in cases with secondary autistic behaviors. This therefore does not differentiate secondary types of ASD.

At the same time, many prior conditions like Rett's syndrome and fragile X are being taken out of the ASD, therefore the numbers of idiopathic cases should be going down. Identification of the other medical diagnoses are not often used in school administrative statistics, and there has been the argument that to get more services the diagnosis is being used more freely. This, however, runs counter to school budgets and state early intervention programs that lack resources and therefore do not want to over-label the problem. Also many commercial insurance programs in most states look at autism as congenital and do not cover medical or ancillary care without resistance. The errors mentioned in the above paragraph would favor an autism diagnosis decline if prior genetic and metabolic cases (such as children with phenylketonuria (PKU) or succinic semialdehyde dehydrogenase deficiency (SSADH) deficiency, Angelman syndrome, or fragile X) are being diagnosed more accurately. So to claim better psychological diagnostic abilities alone as the reason for the increase in the numbers is misleading, because more accuracy in medical diagnoses should also decrease the number of idiopathic cases of ASD. This confusion and seemingly astronomical increase from 1:2500 births in the 1980s to the current Center for Disease Control (CDC) estimate of 1:142 births has led to understandable panic and fear among parents of children with ASD.

There has been no change in the incidence of cerebral palsy for instance in comparison. Mental retardation and other conditions may be decreasing, not because of many children now being labeled with autism, but through better obstetric care and fewer parents with larger families; and better genetic screening may have led to decreased risks for mental retardation. Therefore, the argument that the case for better autism diagnosis replacing prior labels seems to underestimate the rates of mental retardation decline that may be occurring. This may not just be a shift in cases from one category to be labeled autistic, but rather an actual decline in mental retardation over the past two decades. Since these are school-based educational data that are the most quoted estimates, there may be highly inaccurate accounting of other medical conditions that have autistic features. Also relying only on school data may overestimate true autism, as many school districts prefer an autism label in order to provide better programming funding. Recent debates in medical articles on the nature of the diagnostic shift as being responsible quote different rates of autism spectrum cases that are far lower than current estimates provided by the Center for Disease Control that estimates 1:142 births (7:1000 births). Many Department of Education statistics rate an incidence of only 3:1000 births. Any comparison should use individual state programs for educational enrollment instead of the federal estimates as individual state figures for education may be more accurate as well.

The final issue is that there are strong arguments from some academic psychologists using statistical methods to argue against an autism epidemic. These arguments do not seem to match the experience of most current child neurologists. To gain perspective on that, at a meeting of the Child Neurology Society in 2005, there were almost no participants who stood when asked how many cases of autism they personally knew of 10 to 20 years ago, but almost the entire room stood when asked in the past few years how many doctors regularly treated or knew of someone with autism. Clinicians see changes in the rate of this disorder, and the argument that child neurologists and psychiatrists in clinical practice cannot distinguish mental retardation and learning disabilities from autism is a weak argument in my opinion.

These perceived increases, whether factual or not, have led many parents to seek alternative care out of fear of an underlying epidemic. Traditional medicine, mainly in the hands of the developmental pediatric or psychiatry and psychology departments of hospitals and medical centers, has spent most of the past 20 years labeling, but offering little in the way of medical intervention and treatment. This has led to many theories and probable misinterpretations of the causes of autism, as well as misinterpreting the facts that were clinically present as causative for the condition. Many parent groups have taken an anti-medicine approach, or have blamed vaccinations for the rise in autism. However, other support groups have done a more scientifically supportive job. Parent groups like the National Alliance for Autism Research (NAAR) and Cure Autism Now (CAN) raised funds for true genetic and other medical research to move forward. The true understanding of the scope of this problem is just recently being covered by the media, and one media executive has taken up the cause with his own support network called Autism Speaks. All of these efforts and previous foundations by famous sports or movie industry families are all steps in the right direction. Until 2002, very little government support for autism medical research was being done, except in areas utilizing behavioral therapies, with most of the other funds going towards genetic research. Very few double-blind, placebo-controlled treatment-oriented research studies have been done. Yet for parents, treatment-oriented research would be more helpful to guide physicians in the field in neurology, psychiatry, and pediatrics to have a better plan to help alleviate the difficulties that children and families go through from ASD.

This void has again opened the door for parents to waste time and money on therapies and theories that do not work. Many parents resist trusting traditional medicine because they (falsely) believe vaccinations caused their child to get sick in the first place. This delays appropriate referrals for medical evaluation at age 12 to 24 months, with children going instead to occupational or speech or play therapies. The message to parents has been why not try non-medical care or vitamin treatments first. The real importance of treating a brain that is sick, biochemically malfunctioning, perhaps having an immunologically driven regression, or having epileptic activity at night, has not been fostered within the medical community. Medical intervention should be working with these children in the first two years of life. Therapy would certainly go better if medical intervention was done first, or at least simultaneously. I use the example of Alzheimer's disease. If grandma starts to act in repetitive and oversensitive ways, stops sleeping, or stops talking, do you think the family is going to call the park district recreation program, a speech therapist, a physical therapist? Or do you think they will seek out a competent medical doctor, such as a neurologist trained in dementia diagnosis and treatment? This is the state we are in with ASD. We cannot be certain about regression, early development, or causes of ASD if referrals to appropriate medical care specialists are delayed. Early interventional speech and educational supportive therapies are good, but many of my families knew that and still their child did not benefit until medical care was sought. Even then, this remains a chronic and currently incurable condition. We are not yet sure how to prevent ASD either. This leads me to discuss theoretical reasons for the increase in the following chapters. I will focus on the alternative lay beliefs that vaccinations, or wheat/gluten/milk allergy, yeast infection, or mercury poisoning cause autism initially. I will then hypothesize on more medically plausible theories, including various immune theories. Then I will postulate a way to synthesize these apparently diverse ideas and see if any unifying theory may exist. This may be a classic case of the "blind men and the elephant," with different interpretations describing some truth, yet missing it as a whole.

My own bias is to believe that ASD as a whole is increasing in frequency. There is no way to deny the facts of the clinician observations, although statistically the rise may not be as great as the highest numbers quoted. Also the lack of coherence from educational, insurance, and medical sources of information may reflect differing priorities of diagnosis. The official medical community does not yet concede that autism rates are increasing. Many factors discussed in subsequent chapters may offer theoretical clues but no definite answers as to the possible causative factors. It is my hope that future research will help resolve the questions we will raise and discuss.

Chapter 11

Vaccinations, Mercury, and Autism

Public fears of the astronomical rise in diagnosing autistic spectrum disorders (ASD) in children have led to fears that a vaccination, particularly the MMR (measles-mumps-rubella) vaccine, is linked to ASD. Parents are also concerned that a rise seemed to occur at the same time as the guidelines for vaccinations changed in the early 1990s to increase the available number of required vaccines and compress these within the first 15 months of life. The first newer vaccine protecting against haemophilus influenza meningitis was introduced in the late 1980s. Hepatitis B vaccinations were added for routine newborn vaccination due to public policy to eradicate an increasing risk of this disease especially in urban poor and immigrant areas. This became a series of three vaccines at birth, two months, and then at 12 to 15 months. At the same time the MMR was moved from 18 to 24 months to 12 to 15 months. These changes coincidentally parallel the time when ASD increases have been noted. Some parents have tried hard to link these. More paranoia began when a report came out suggesting a possible MMR link to Crohn's disease. Then in 1998, Wakefield published an article in the British journal *The Lancet* that tried to link the MMR to autistic regression and intestinal lymphoid hyperplasia (essentially lymph node enlargement in the intestine, like tonsils getting enlarged in the throat). In a very small series of autistic children, and later describing measles ribonucleic acid (RNA) fragments found in autistic children's intestines, Wakefield and his colleagues claimed this linked the MMR to autism. This has also been described in normal patients and there is yet to be duplication at another research site. Later the majority of co-authors of Wakefield's report retracted their belief that the report conclusively linked the findings to autism. The claimed relationship from Wakefield's initial observations that MMR vaccines caused a new form of colitis and that some types of ASD evolve from this has also not been substantiated. In fact, the majority of co-authors of Wakefield's original paper linking ileal lymphoid hyperplasia to ASD retracted their implied agreement on the explanation of the findings. Although ASD children may appear to suffer from higher rates of gastroesophageal reflux, perhaps more intestinal inflammation, and constipation, lactose intolerance, and diarrhea than their typically developing peers, there is no firm evidence that a direct linkage to the MMR exists. In fact, other developmental disorders also have high rates of constipation, gastroesophageal reflux, and other eating disorders as well. The danger of not vaccinating against measles may certainly lead to a measles epidemic, and 1:1000 children may go on to suffer severe neurological injury from direct measles infection, not to mention the rubella and mumps morbidity that would also increase. Autistic outcomes have also resulted directly from measles infection.

Shortly after the theory of MMR-induced autism arose, the theory of exposure to cumulative amounts of mercury was put forward as the cause of increased incidence in ASD rather than a direct measles effect. Proponents of this theory believed that children developed ASD from mercury poisoning through exposure to biologically unavailable mercury in the form of thimerosal preservative in many vaccines. Even though these vaccines and thimerosal contained a biologically non-absorbable form of mercury (ethyl-mercury), parents and some public figures continued to support this postulation. This led to public hearings and worldwide reviews and research into vaccine safety.

The result of this controversial belief and fear was to review data from many countries to analyze the rate of ASD compared to vaccination schedules, as well as review known mercury exposure risks, and also to compare data where mercury-free vaccines were available. Retrospective population data were analyzed in Japan, Finland, Great Britain, the United States, Denmark, and Sweden. These studies found no link between MMR and ASD or gastrointestinal diseases. Mercury available in thimerosal was in the form of ethyl-mercury, not the methyl mercury found in seafood, or other biological environmental poisonings. High seafood diets in pregnant women exposed to methyl mercury were found to present no risk in a published study from the Seychelles Islands looking at prenatal exposure and subsequent rate of ASD. However, another study in a different location where high percentages of whale meat is consumed found higher prenatal mercury correlating to more birth defects and abnormal development. The maximal elemental amount of exposure to mercury (not necessarily biologically absorbable) was 187.5 micrograms prior to 1999, but after the vaccines in the United States became mercury-free from thimerosal after 2001, the exposure was 3 micrograms. Despite this decrease in mercury, there is still an apparently overall increasing incidence of ASD being diagnosed as per 2007 statistics collected by the State of California as one source looking at educational and regional center enrollment.

A thorough review by the Institute of Medicine was published in 2004. This review of vaccine safety concluded that there was no reason to change the current vaccination schedule owing to ASD risk from thimerosal, but did suggest removing it where possible as a precaution. The committee also recommended carefully controlled research for chelation claims, and that future research was needed regarding the claims of alternative practitioners relative to chelation. Recent data from the MIND Institute at the University of California Davis campus showed no baseline differences in autistic children from controls regarding mercury or other heavy metals in their screening as part of the CHARGE study. Danish studies looking at thimerosal-preserved and thimerosal-free vaccines and comparing rates of ASD came to the conclusion that thimerosal did not increase the rate of ASD in the Danish population. The committee from the Institute of Medicine finally found no causal relationship between thimerosal-containing vaccines and ASD. As time goes on since thimerosal-free vaccines have been given, the mercury theory should be shown to be incorrect. There is no current logic that chelation actually has any direct effect for this reason. In my 16 years treating children with ASD, I have seen no controlled research published in the medical literature documenting claims made by chelation doctors. No actively chelating doctor has any current research that is being published showing pre- and post-treatment controlled results. Also no patient by hair, urine, or blood testing has shown pre- or post-treatment evidence that any mercury poisoning ever existed. The use of chelation skin sprays makes no sense at all in my medical opinion.

Recently, a group from Columbia University in New York published a mouse study of a genetic strain at risk for autoimmune problems exposed to levels of thimerosal mimicking exposure seen in infants prior to 2001. This mouse genetic strain has no known human equivalent immune defect at the current time. This research did show autoimmune defense changes in the animals after thimerosal exposure and changes in their behaviors that had some resemblance to autistic features. This study is important as a possible model for environmental changes causing autistic features in a population subgroup that may have greater risk than normally expected, yet cannot be directly assumed at this time to explain what exactly has happened in human cases of ASD. It does not conclude exactly which component of thimerosal versus genetic factor is responsible for the changes observed. Also it may not be the mercury but another chemical trigger on the mouse's immune system that did the damage observed. Some prior immune studies have also suggested that some autoimmune factors on T-cells can be altered by exposure to ethyl mercury to increase interleukin 2 levels and trigger an autoimmune cascade. Again this has not been widely studied.

There has been some more research in mice suggesting that thimerosal may injure cellular function in neuronal cell lines where potential release of certain cytokines may alter dendrites that make connections between nerve cells that may alter inter-neuronal communication. This may alter the neuroglial immune cells and how they interact. Caution in interpretation is required here as this was a study in cell lines not in an animal brain, and certain neuronal cells in a living animal may not react the same way as this laboratory cell culture model. Also different cell lines may respond differently and to different doses in this research. However, this may represent that certain patients could be more sensitive to environmental factors such as thimerosal. Newer theories from several universities including the University of California Davis and Johns Hopkins University have shown both immune and environmental factors that potentially relate to autism, including recent findings of pesticide exposure increasing risks in those exposed during pregnancy within 500 feet of spraying of pesticide in central California. The evidence as of 2007 shows no single causative agent, and since thimerosal exposure has now declined this should be less of a future issue in the search for causation.

The devil's advocate position to all this is that there may be some as yet undetermined injury that has led to increased rates of ASD related to vaccinations. One theory is that vaccinations since the 1950s to current times have saved some susceptible children with poor immune resistance to these deadly childhood illnesses. This combined with multitudes of improved antibiotic coverage for frequent childhood infections such as otitis media (inner ear infection), pneumonia, and streptococcal infections may have also led to a different genetic pool that has reproduced over the last 50 years. This means more children may be born with immune susceptibility to acquired serious infections, or may have altered immune response to current infections, modification of such infections by antibiotics, or altered immune response brought on by vaccination, or a combination of these effects. Perhaps 1:100 may evoke an inflammatory autoimmune response that could attack brain, vascular, or intestinal sites leading to some features seen in ASD subgroups with infection. Another possible theory centers on the change in the number and types of vaccines infants were exposed to after 1991 compared to the preceding immunization schedule. At that time, there was the addition of a neonatal hepatitis B vaccine, and the subsequent hepatitis B injections, along with an earlier MMR and the addition of the haemophilus influenza (HiBB) vaccine. Theoretically, certain children may have an aberrant shift of their developing and immature immune system to become primed for a predominantly autoimmune response that alters neuronal connections due to inflammatory disruption of neurogenesis or synaptic formation. This theory would require looking not at thimerosal or MMR, but at the total vaccination exposure, and also looking more specifically at the newer vaccine requirements, specifically hepatitis B, HiBB, and MMR timing in relation to the increasing rate of ASD diagnosis since 1991. To the best of my knowledge this has not yet been done in this way.

The take-home message for this chapter is that there is no definitive causation linking vaccination directly to the apparent rise in cases of autism. There may be environmental factors that alter the innate central nervous system immune response, and this research is just beginning to be done. Possible overstressing of immature immune systems that are susceptible to autoimmune alterations may be part of what goes wrong as a possible trigger or mechanism for autism and other ASD cases. Not vaccinating our children is also risky for many lethal or potentially developmentally impairing infections. Parents should discuss rationally with their pediatricians the safest way to immunize their children. There is currently not enough medical evidence from the real scientific community to support that vaccination or thimerosal has caused the current autism epidemic. Also remember that for most vaccinations since 2001 to 2002, thimerosal is no longer used in the United States and most other developed countries.

Chapter 12

Immunology and Autoimmunity
Is There a Causative Relationship with Autistic Spectrum Disorders?

Autoimmune disease refers to dysfunction of a person's immune system such that the immune response attacks its own body tissues. Many diseases exist that meet this definition. Neurological diseases include giant cell arteritis, multiple sclerosis, Guillain-Barre syndrome, myasthenia gravis, and opsoclonus-myoclonus. Neurological diseases that may have an autoimmune component include Alzheimer's disease, amyotrophic lateral sclerosis (Lou Gehrig's disease), Parkinson's disease, and now theoretically some types of autism. Systemic autoimmune diseases that can affect the nervous system include systemic lupus erythematosis (SLE), rheumatoid arthritis, Hashimoto's thyroiditis, Crohn's disease, and many others. Certain infections can also yield autoimmune responses that affect the nervous system: chicken pox can lead to varicella cerebellar demyelination, and post-streptococcal group A infection sequellae include Syndenham's chorea and, perhaps less-known, PANDAS (post-streptococcal autoimmune neurological disease syndrome) with obsessive-compulsive or tic-like behaviors. These known cross-reactive immune-driven attacks on the nervous system can have various degrees of severity. The exact role in autism is currently unknown but being studied.

History of autoimmune disease and autism

Initial observation of some family histories when children had autism had revealed a higher than normal incidence of maternal or familial autoimmune diseases such as Hashimoto's thyroiditis, Crohn's disease, SLE, and other diseases. Some researchers, such as the late Reed Warren, noted certain genetic markers called HLA haplotypes typically associated with autoimmune disease to be associated with increased rates of autism in families with autoimmune histories. Interestingly, diseases such as asthma and multiple sclerosis are not frequently associated with autistic spectrum disorders (ASD); however, a recent report from pregnant mothers with asthma did show a higher risk for ASD in offspring. This may be due to some asthma treatments these mothers were exposed to and not just having asthma. Occasional reports of immune studies in groups of children with autism have shown evidence of antibodies being produced that could cause potential autoimmune damage or reflect that type of autoimmune reaction within the children studied. Some researchers noted in the 1990s an apparent increased rate of otitis media or frequent upper respiratory disease in up to 70 percent of their patients diagnosed with autism. This led to reports of a higher than expected rate of lower levels of immunoglobulins IgG, IgA, or IgG subclasses compared to normal controls in 30 percent of children with ASD. These observations led to two published treatment protocols with intravenous immunoglobulin therapy with a 10 percent response rate in autism behavioral improvement by two different researchers. There were also published case reports about children responding to steroid treatment. The exact mechanism of steroid response in epilepsy and ASD is still not fully understood. There is a belief that anti-inflammatory effects are a mechanism of steroid action in these conditions. Although earlier pathology reports did not show inflammatory changes, and very infrequent studies of cerebrospinal fluid were done in the past, more recent studies have been done that challenge that observation from initial anatomy studies in autism.

Recent studies of autoimmune evidence in autism

More recent studies have reported the presence of anti-endothelial antibodies that may cross-react against capillary endothelial cells (perhaps from small blood vessel inflammation or vasculitis in the brain at the capillary level), anti-neuronal antibodies, and antibodies against Brain-Derived Neurotrophic Factor (BDNF). These anti-endothelial antibodies were either IgG or IgM types (Figure 12.1). These were not observed in normal controls, but more in ASD patients, as well as severe epileptic syndromes such as Lennox-Gastaut types, some autoimmune children with rheumatoid arthritis, and children with Landau-Kleffner syndrome. Therefore these antibodies were not very specific. There have also been noted increases of antibodies against gliadin (a marker for wheat/gluten sensitivity), but usually of the IgG type in children with ASD, not the IgA type which is seen in celiac disease. These anti-gliadin IgG subtypes of ASD children do not have clinical celiac disease. The presence of serum antibodies against myelin basic protein have been reported, but recent lumbar puncture results in one study do not show elevation of myelin basic protein in the cerebrospinal fluid. Other authors reported possible immune markers against certain T-cell surface antibodies like CD 26, and also questionable presence of antibodies against casein and gluten protein-like cross-reactions towards certain T-cell receptors. These studies are interesting, but do not prove a specific strong cause and effect of these antibodies, but merely the possibility of an over-reactive and dysfunctional immune system.

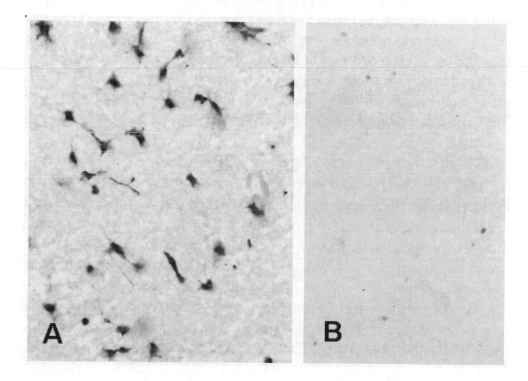

Figure 12.1: Serum anti-endothelial antibodies against brain capillary endothelial cells from patient serum with ASD and regression (A); staining is not seen in control patient without ASD (B)

More impressive links to an immune role in autism have been published. First is the data derived from the large study of cord blood samples taken from over 800 infants, and then looking at the presence of certain markers in the group of children that went on to develop autism, compared to normal controls, and another group with mental retardation or cerebral palsy. One such protein was BDNF again and, among others, macrophage chemoattractant protein (MCP-1). There were definite markers for an intrauterine insult of autoimmune, infectious, or hypoxic type in children with autism or cerebral palsy, but not in isolated mental retardation or normal controls. Recent research at Johns Hopkins Hospital has shown the presence of neuroglial activation and elevated MCP-1 levels, as well as other neuroglial derived cytokines in 11 brain samples from patients with autism. The same authors reported cerebrospinal fluid elevation of cytokines including MCP-1 and interleukin 6. Interestingly, recent epilepsy models are showing how cytokine inflammatory responses are pro-epileptic and elevated in epileptic tissue. BDNF may influence certain receptor types such as N-methyl-D-aspartate (NMDA) receptors and also promotes neuronal hyper-excitability in central nervous system cell types. BDNF mRNA (messenger RNA that is produced by the cell nucleus to produce the protein) is increased at sites of epileptogenesis. BDNF may promote epileptogenesis by its effect on the tyrosine kinase B receptor, which in turn acts upon gamma-aminobutyric acid (GABA)-ergic and glutamatergic receptors. A recent mouse model of Rett's syndrome has implicated there may be deficient BDNF protein, and manipulation of increased BDNF modifies the Rett's-type symptoms.

Glutamate may play an end-stage role in cellular damage invoked in certain autoimmune and cytokine activated neuroinflammatory responses. Glutamate increases Tumor Necrosis Factor-alpha (TNF-α) and TNF-α may be elevated in spinal fluid compared to serum levels in autistic children with regression in one small study recently performed. One mouse model of SLE shows that anti-deoxyribonucleic acid (DNA) antibodies cross-react with NMDA receptors that modulate glutamate and can mediate cellular excitotoxicity and damage. This is yet another model of a possible mechanism that could also happen in subtypes of ASD and regression. As mentioned earlier, anti-capillary and brain endothelial antibodies from serum are elevated in certain epilepsy types, Landau- Kleffner syndrome (LKS), and also ASD. These antibodies also react against BDNF.

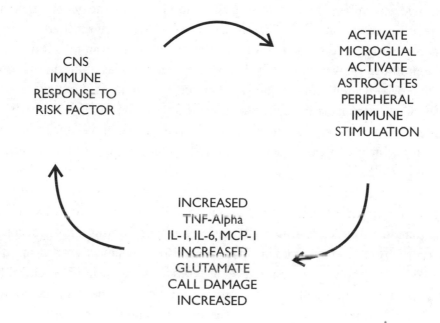

Figure 12.2: Central nervous system (CNS) immune activation response

These separate research observations are therefore starting to coalesce into a more unified group of potentially relevant information. As seen in Figure 12.2, an interactive potential model would be a central nervous system or brain exposure to some combination of intrauterine or postnatal exposure that triggers a neuroglial reaction that then releases a cascade of immune factors like cytokines or cellular immune responses that then alter neuronal signaling or connectivity and may cause abnormal central nervous system response. This can become self-perpetuating as well. Theoretical predisposition or sensitivity to this type of central nervous system immune response may differentiate those prone to autism from those who are not.

Immunizations and autism

The fact that abnormal immune responses are being observed in ASD patients clinically as well as from brain tissue, spinal fluid, and serum samples from these patients, begs the question as to how these children respond to immunizations. No one currently has looked at predisposing risk factors that may put some sub-groups of children at risk for the current schedule and at types of national immunization policies in place in most modern countries. These policies are designed assuming everyone in the population has the same general risk factors for reacting to vaccinations. Therefore, no one really knows if there are specific tests that could predict the risk of an adverse immunization reaction. Actually, the fears raised have only really focused on the measles, mumps, and rubella vaccine (MMR), and unfortunately on mercury content of shots given prior to 2001. Current vaccination changes have eliminated the ethyl-mercury risk from thimerosal. The exact biological risk and levels of mercury damage for methyl mercury typically found in seafood or environmental spills is known. The exact amount of ethyl-mercury that really is biologically a danger or even absorbed from thimerosal preservatives is still not clear. From the past 15 years of practice and reviewing the literature, I have seen no convincing medical observation or data that any child with ASD really has mercury poisoning. This is because the alternative practitioners who do hair analysis or chelation with urine testing have failed to show in any patient records I have seen, or in the medical literature, even a single well-documented case report of mercury poisoning in children with autism treated with chelation. This and the reviews of the Center for Disease Control, and the recent report from the Institute of Medicine, confirm a lack of a statistically meaningful link to the MMR vaccine, as well as no evidence to link mercury to ASD. Many reports from other countries, including the United Kingdom, Finland, Japan, and Denmark, show that the MMR is not linked to ASD. There is further evidence from Denmark that vaccines with and without thimerosal have similar low risk to cause ASD. The recommendations from all of the controversy have led to a change in removing thimerosal from infant vaccinations since 2001 in the United States, and yet the rate of ASD continues to rise. This over time should dispel the false belief that mercury poisoning causes ASD, and that chelation has any beneficial role.

One criticism of the reviews on vaccination is the failure actually to look at the types of viral and bacterial immunizations that are given, and perhaps at the timing of vaccinations that changed in 1991. At that time hepatitis B vaccine was added as a required vaccination at birth to two weeks, two months and one year, and the MMR was moved back from age two years to 12 to 15 months. This was done as a public policy measure with the worthy goal of eliminating hepatitis B from the general population. The increased frequency and compression of the vaccination schedule was designed to help compliance with the vaccination and well child care promoted by the American Academy of Pediatrics. The rates of ASD have dramatically risen since this time. It is possible that, because of successful infectious disease interventions since the 1940s, more people are alive and reproducing who have impaired immune systems. Antibiotics and vaccinations have decreased infant mortality and allowed more people to survive to reproductive potential over the last two generations than ever before in history. The question is whether this has led to a more susceptible or dysfunctional subgroup that may have a higher risk of an autoimmune or abnormal immune response to infections or immunizations. There may be infants where the immune system may get primed the wrong way, especially if too early in infancy. Exposure may trigger some degree of autoimmune reaction. There may be intrauterine factors as well, as implied by the study showing cord blood factors that suggest intrauterine infectious, ischemic, or autoimmune markers in autistic children. The future research questions for ASD and vaccination as an environmental factor should focus on exposure to the timing and types of vaccinations used since 1991. The theoretical idea is that vaccinations or certain infections may act upon a predisposed genetic immune risk factor, lead to inflammatory glial changes, neuronal growth or interconnectivity disruption, and then eventual regression or loss of skills that lead to core symptoms of autism. This would fit into the complex heterogeneous population that is seen in ASD.

Conclusion

This chapter has focused on the newest research in ASD, especially related to the role of autoimmunity and vaccination in the etiology of the current observed increased incidence of these disorders. Subsequent chapters will focus on the treatment of ASD core symptoms, and the potential for autoimmune therapy to modulate or perhaps change the course of ASD will be discussed. There is no immediate answer on whether a change in immunization schedules or some other factor would decrease the risk for ASD. One suggestion would be to randomize a group of infants without known immediate risk for hepatitis B, and give one group the current schedule, with the other group not getting the MMR until age two or three years, and holding the hepatitis B until age three to five years. If there were a difference in the incidence of ASD between the groups, then perhaps the question of immunizations and risk for ASD would be clarified. Complex research questions on the exact role of neuroglial inflammation and neurotrophic factors observed will be understood better in the near future. This offers exciting hope that screening tests and treatments that can modify or reverse ASD will be available.

Chapter 13

Theories on a Prenatal Cause

The last two chapters have focused on theories of immunizations and immunological factors as potential causes of autistic spectrum disorder (ASD). There are other theories which are based on neuroanatomical and genetic findings. The exact role of these different theoretical models is unclear. The debate of predetermined versus acquired disorder continues at this time.

Prenatal determination of autism

The fact that two thirds of ASD do not regress and seem present from early infancy makes a strong argument for a predetermined or prenatal onset. There is good evidence to support that perhaps the majority of ASD subtypes are genetic or intrauterine in onset.

The first studies that proposed this possibility were the neuropathology studies of Dr. Margaret Baumen and colleagues from Massachusetts General Hospital at Harvard. These and subsequent brain tissue studies found that abnormal cellular appearance of neurons in the cerebellum, pons, mesial temporal and inferior frontal areas may correspond to an injury that they estimated to occur at around 27 weeks' gestation. This was based on certain neuronal arrangements in the brainstem with regressive findings suggestive of damage at that developmental stage. Other findings that suggest an intrauterine event are perhaps the magnetic resonance imaging (MRI) abnormalities found in the cerebellar regions that may have prenatal origins. More recent anatomical observations of abnormal head circumference growth between birth and two years of age compared to controls suggest an onset after birth later in infancy. There is a possibility that both observations are connected. Unfortunately we do not have data from the brain tissue bank to show that these same children also had rapid head circumference growth in the first two years of life. It is also possible that neuroglial inflammation in utero may cause changes in neuronal formation or neuroplasticity. Recent data suggest that, instead of a lack of development, neuronal cell damage may be the cause of some of the reported cerebellar microscopic changes in Purkinje cells that have previously been described; the retrograde degeneration was caused by a neuro-inflammatory effect, not some pre-programmed prenatal genetic cause. This is obviously an area of debate at this time.

Another argument for intrauterine, possible inflammatory onset of ASD has been published in the examination of markers within the cord blood of over 800 infants in California. These markers were abnormal for children who went on to get the diagnosis of cerebral palsy or autism, yet were normal in mental retardation patients without obvious brain injury. These proteins included markers mentioned in the chapter on immunology including BDNF (Brain-Derived Neurotrophic Factor), VIP (vasopressin intestinal protein), and MAC-1 (macrophage chemoattractant complex). This helps unify with possible infectious, ischemic, or other immunologically driven injury that may occur in the prenatal period. These findings may be a trigger for neurodevelopmental errors in the growth and interconnectivity of neurons. The fact that identification of some of these markers was present at birth may offer a possible screening and intervention strategy that may prevent subsequent alterations to neuronal organization. Perhaps neuroprotective treatments can be designed to correct aberrant autoimmune or abnormal nerve growth factors that signal dysgenesis possibly occurring in the brains of patients with some forms of ASD. There is also recent evidence of a human maternal circulating antibody that attacks fetal rat brain in 11/11 mothers of autistic children, but not from 10/10 control samples. This again suggests a prenatal immune mechanism may play a role in ASD.

Genetics theory

The genetic research described in Chapter 9 also suggests a high degree of genetic predetermination of ASD. For instance, Rett's syndrome and fragile X have a genetic origin, although secondary autistic features arise. The same is true for some animal models of autism. Many genes are being studied as having links to ASD, but the role they actually play in the full clinical manifestation of ASD remains unknown. Perhaps these genes, in combination with postnatal or intrauterine events, interact to create a clinical presentation of autism. There is still much work needed to be completed to understand better the role of neurotropic factors, glial cells, and genetics on the development of ASD. There is no unifying gene theory for ASD at this time. In fact the genetic picture emerging is complex and more supportive of a heterogeneous group of disorders with similar clinical manifestations. In the future, genotypic subtypes may be helpful in screening for possible treatment responses. For instance, if a defect for serotonin or dopamine production is present, or a risk for autoimmune or epileptic defect is present, preventive or restorative treatments may be more easily designed. Also a better understanding of genetic susceptibility to environmental factors can be determined.

Biochemical theories of autism

The observation of certain patterns of repetitive and ritualistic behaviors in autism has led to theories of biochemical defects. There are some diseases with errors in biochemistry that may mimic autism. One such is Smith-Lemli-Opitz disease, where a defect in cholesterol metabolism is noted to coincide with some autistic behaviors unless treated. Phenylketonuria and hypothyroidism may have overlapping features of autism if untreated, but usually present more as retardation.

Early theories of the role of serotonin led to treatment studies that theorized increasing serotonin would help symptoms of autism, but these studies have provided limited help. A theory of neonatal exposure to pitocin (a drug used to induce uterine contractions hormonally in labor) has led to treatment trials with oxytocin (the hormone that is produced during labor) that have yielded some social improvements, yet do not prove a true link to a cause of autism. There are positron emission tomography (PET) scan studies showing changes in serotonin metabolism over the lifespan in autistic individuals, yet the exact meaning and etiology of observed patterns remains unclear. Small groups of patients with purine metabolism defects and autism features have been noted, but do not comprise a major subgroup of ASD. These and other observations of some chemical aspects of subgroups with autism may suggest some inherited defect in brain biochemistry.

Chapter 14

Common Alternative Medicine Theories

Most alternative practitioners in the field of autistic spectrum disorders (ASD) have a multitude of theories that they refer to as orthomolecular medicine and the biomedical approach. This is often confusing and misleading to parents as it gives the impression of well-researched and thought-out theories. It is based on the idea that autism is the result of a series of biochemical defects in the central nervous system and that vitamins or minerals would work to straighten out the problem, hence the term "orthomolecular" (to straighten the molecules). There are also theories of gastrointestinal damage and subsequent toxins being absorbed via the intestinal tract. There are also theories on yeast metabolism as a causative factor in autism. This is the same culture that gave rise to chelation therapy for presumed mercury poisoning and false hope for secretin therapy as well as promoting the gluten-/casein-free diet.

Alternative biochemical theories

This is the work promoted by supporters of high-dose vitamin supplementation, mostly known as orthomolecular theory. This focuses on certain biological pathways called methylation affecting dopaminergic and B6 and folic acid pathways in the Krebs metabolic cycle for brain energy and neurotransmitter production. They have over the years made claims for high doses of vitamin B6, magnesium, dimethylglycine (DMG), and, more recently, methylcobalamine injections (methyl B12) to promote methylation, and also glutathione to promote anti-oxidant protection.

Biochemically this is based on a theory that there may be an error in cysteine, homocysteine, and methionine, which DMG is supposed to help to normalize. Vitamin B12 in the form of methyl B12 may play a role here. The idea behind this is that the abnormal methylation of cysteine leads to a bio-chemical blockage of precursors to certain neurotransmitters including dopamine and serotonin. This defect is also theorized to play a role in the anti-oxidative stress that leads to free radical damage. This has been tied to recent studies suggesting glutathione is lower in autistic children vs. controls. Proponents of these theories suppose that all ASD subtypes are similar in bio-chemical nature of the defect, and all should respond to a cookie-cutter approach that includes a mixture of a multiple supplement treatment that in essence should enhance the conversion of cysteine and homocysteine to methionine and glutathione. These same proponents have adapted the mercury toxicity theory on the basis that heavy metals increase oxidative stress and use up excess glutathione, and also that it would interfere with this methyl B12 activity causing a functional deficiency in available methyl B12.

At this time there are no controlled studies to support these claims, nor are there good clinical ways to measure these proposed biochemical defects. Also it is unclear, even if you correct for anti-oxidant protection factors, that this would enhance appropriate neuroprotection, create better balances of neurotransmitters, or lead to improved function. Certainly increasing anti-oxidant protection can help in a number of neurological diseases, but there may be better ways to do this than the current array of vitamins, injections, chelation, and other complex regimens offered by practitioners who believe in this theory.

In light of the increasing scientific observations being made in the genetics, immunological, and neuroimaging of ASD, these biochemical alternative treat-ment theories may represent at best a cofactor that is under stress in the complex brain dysfunction seen in ASD. It is also possible that immune stressors can delete anti-oxidant protection mechanisms from chronic inflammation. There are no published controlled studies on any of these treatments. One child died from intravenous chelation due to calcium depletion. Although the proponents said it was a pharmacy error, the real question is why is chelation being done with no scientific reason to justify the treatment? This is the problem when medically trying to help parents confused by these alternative practitioners promising cures based only on anecdotal theories and testimonials. If the chelation, B12 injections, or glutathione treatments being done have any merit, it may be at the level of anti-oxidant protection. At this time, there is no scientific merit to this potentially harmful therapy. Also high rates of hyperactivity occur with B12 injections in patients with autism. Chelation can harm liver and kidneys, and remove some essential metals such as iron and calcium. There is no evidence that skin creams or sprays have any biological effect for chelation or glutathione replenishment.

Gastrointestinal and yeast theories

In addition to complex biochemical theories, there have been a number of alternative theories on the role of intestinal dysfunction, casein, wheat, and possible yeast metabolites as a causative factor in autism. The role of gastrointestinal dysfunction is debatable since most of these theories are based without any diagnostic work-up of the intestinal tract. There has only recently been an increasing trend for gastroenterologists to take complaints from the autism population seriously. This has been the case in the past for other neuropsychiatric disorders. There are real findings of increased constipation and pseudo-diarrhea from the blockage. This is called encoporesis or stool retention. This is seen in a number of other neurologic conditions including attention deficit disorder, cerebral palsy, and obsessive-compulsive disorder. There is evidence of increased lactose intolerance as well. There is very poor evidence of increased celiac disease or intolerance to gluten in this population by either serum studies or endoscopic proof. In fact when studied, celiac sprue is rarely found. When this rare disease is treated in ASD, intestinal symptoms may clear up but the autism is not better. There is no evidence to date that the intestines of these children are injured thereby allowing passage of toxic substances into the bloodstream and brain, the so-called "leaky gut." There is no evidence of an opioid-like toxic effect from wheat or milk metabolites affecting these children with ASD. In fact studies of opioid blockers have not successfully changed clinical features in the autism population to a significant degree. The majority of children tested by actual skin sensitivity or serum blood tests with Food and Drug Administration (FDA)-approved laboratory tests do not show any allergy to milk or wheat. Many believers in the intestinal theories suggest the gluten/casein-free diet. In 15 years of practice, even with actual comorbid diagnosis of true milk or wheat allergy or celiac disease, this author has not seen a significant improvement in autistic behaviors, even if intestinal discomfort may improve. Can certain immune factors on certain T-cell receptors possibly be mediated by anti-gluten allergic type antibodies? This possibility of an effect on the immune system is possibly another small medical risk for some patients with ASD who are cross-reactive to gluten or wheat. However, a genetic predisposition must coexist.

Yeast metabolites are another theory that produces toxic brain effects. One strong proponent of this theory promoted urine tests for so-called yeast metabolites. In one randomized study with antibiotic treatment, no difference from controls was observed in the urine tested in this fashion. Many patients have tried systemic yeast treatments. There is no evidence in any patient with autism of systemic yeast infection. Stool cultures cannot accurately show yeast infection due to errors of aerobic collection that kill the majority of normal anaerobic bacteria and therefore allow yeast or other bacteria to overgrow in samples mailed to these alternative laboratories. Therefore there is no reason to support the yeast theory in autism as a major factor in the etiology of ASD.

PART IV
Treating Autistic Spectrum Disorders

Chapter 15

Overview of Treatment

There is a great need for improving the quality of life for children and adults with autistic spectrum disorders (ASD). Although there are agreed upon diagnostic standards, and as previously shown recommendations from several areas of medicine suggesting medical evaluations that should be done, there are currently no recommended algorithms for treating this devastating condition. This makes it difficult for parents to decide which medications are appropriate for their child, and who to believe. At this time there are still the proverbial "snake oil salesmen" promising cures and "cookie cutter" treatments. There are limited research studies with just a few small controlled studies which are mainly aimed at some core symptoms of ASD, but do not yet offer cures. This is frustrating for medical professionals as well as families living with ASD.

The medical mainstream is coming slowly to grips with autism and pervasive developmental disorder (PDD) conditions which remain lifelong yet not life-shortening. The estimated cost, based on separate studies from Massachusetts Institute of Technology (MIT) and the United Kingdom, for raising an average autistic child from birth to 70 years is approximately $3.5 to 4 million per child, 90 percent of which is for supportive treatment and medical care, with 10 percent the basic needs of food and shelter. This is remarkable economic burden for our society as a whole. This is why it is critical to find medical treatments that would allow better functioning of language and behavior, and in the future reversal of some or all symptoms.

The medical profession is currently under siege by insurance companies at many levels. Many promising drug therapies for ASD may be or usually are "off label" use. This means the Food and Drug Administration (FDA) in the United States, and similar agencies in other countries, have not approved a particular medicine for use in ASD or for use in children, for example. Insurance companies might not pay for such drugs, or might not hassle doctors for approval documentation for their patients to get the drug. Newer drugs can be very expensive. Also due to rising malpractice insurance and medical-legal problems for physicians, many doctors may be afraid to try new or unusual medicine applications for ASD without the approval of the FDA, or in the absence of medical literature that shows with proper research that the treatments are safe, with a low risk to high benefit ratio, and that they treat some symptoms of ASD effectively. This resistance slows progress to try new things. This may limit how many patients with ASD can get new drug trials as some doctors may only try things as part of research studies, if at all.

Another problem defining what works for ASD is that researchers do not have great tools to monitor changes in this condition. There are currently no cures, so outcomes focus on global behavioral improvement, less irritability or less anxiety. Most studies have not accurately focused on core language or social deficits. This should not be an insurmountable obstacle in the future as methods are being improved for research measurements. Many parents also do not live in a vacuum with these children and fluctuations in environment and normal growth and developmental changes may sometimes cause an apparent placebo effect, or a drug might appear to have a side-effect. An example would be a change in teacher or an aide at school causing an apparent increase in irritability and increased tantrums at school, but the child's parents interpret this as a medication effect. The apparent positive placebo effect is higher also because many changes in treating ASD are subjectively measured. There may be a 10 to 30 percent placebo effect. This requires a larger number of children and better controlled studies both of which slow progress and increase the expense of doing the research.

Despite these discouraging facts, there are now better funding, more organizations, and better medications for ASD than at any time in the past. This is why this book is attempting to bring parents up to date on what medications are useful in comorbid symptoms of ASD. Risperdal is now approved by the FDA for autism and there may be one or two further drugs that will be approved by 2010. This does not mean there is a lack of experience with many medications to help behaviors or symptoms of ASD that the following chapters will discuss.

In concluding this introduction for treatment, let me emphasize this truth. This book is a map for parents and medical professionals to learn quickly what drugs have been tried, for what reason, with what outcome, and when to think about using these drugs. As a child neurologist writing this book, I am going to be as objective as possible. I cannot possibly eliminate all of my own clinical experience, nor would I want to, as this may allow sharing of information for my colleagues. I do not want anyone to think that the following chapters are officially sanctioned as a treatment regimen or recommendation by any official medical society or organization at this time. In fact, I hope this book will open discussion between parents and physicians to choose appropriate medications individually for a given child with ASD. This book is not a "cookbook" and I am not recommending this as a prescription for any one of these drugs. This is merely a template to think about ASD from a medication treatment prospective to improve quality of life for these patients. Readers must still base treatment on their own physician's recommendations and experience.

Chapter 16

Choosing a Physician

What is a child neurologist?

A child neurologist is a specialist trained in general pediatrics for two to three years, then having three years of neurology training in adult and child neurology. They are often board-certified in both pediatrics and child neurology. Some have additional training in further specialty areas such as this author has had in epilepsy. Unfortunately child neurologists who are board-certified comprise around 1100 physicians in the United States at this time. Other pediatric specialists such as a developmental pediatricians, child psychiatrists, or even well-trained general pediatricians can often do an adequate neurological medical history and examination if they have had proper training. If no child neurologist is available, then question the comfort level and prior experience of your physician in performing a general neurology exam in children.

What is a developmental pediatrician?

A developmental pediatrician is a physician who trains three years in general pediatrics and then one to two years in a developmental pediatric specialty program emphasizing developmental and school delays. They are not trained in electroencephalography (EEG), but in many programs get some neurology exposure. The American Academy of Pediatric Specialties and the Child Neurology Society have been working to unify training with an overlap with child neurology, and there is a probable future uniting to some degree of the specialties of child neurologists and child developmentalists in the United States. Many times these child development specialists run autism programs, usually more often than child neurologists.

What is a child psychiatrist?

This subspecialty is a person who does six months to a year of general medicine or pediatrics, then does a three-year psychiatry residency and an additional year of child psychiatry. Training has some clinical neurology but no EEG and limited neuroimaging and genetic training. Emphasis is on psychiatric conditions and behavioral conditions. Despite some of these limitations, many child psychiatrists are beginning to be better trained in the neurological and biological basis of conditions such as autism. Again, interviewing a specialist is critical to getting the appropriate level of medical care needed in autism.

General pediatrician/family practitioner

A general pediatrician is trained for three years in pediatrics and may have exposure to some neurological training, and even some minimal autism training, especially in current times. In some communities, general practitioners or family practitioners are the only doctors available for child care. They are trained in most states in a general internal medicine/pediatric based residency program promoting primary care. Both of these types of physicians traditionally have limited training in autistic spectrum disorders (ASD). They can, however, provide medical care for general pediatric illness and make appropriate referrals for medical or psychological testing. They can certainly order all of the medical laboratory, genetic, and many specialized tests in this book. They can also prescribe all medications discussed.

Self-proclaimed autism specialists

There are no standard medical boards or specific training requirements for autism specialists. Most come from one of the first three categories above. There unfortunately have arisen cult-like camps of physicians who practice so-called autism specialty clinics, detoxification practices, "holistic treatments," and other non-recognized treatments without any scientific studies to back them up. Most of these practitioners are not trained specifically in neurology, psychiatry, or developmental pediatrics. In my experience from parental reports, some alternative treatment centers do not even examine the autistic child. In one example of a nationally advertised center in the Chicago area, a physician may not even see the child, only a medical assistant or nurse. These practitioners prey on parental fears and naivety by offering "cookie cutter" or "one size fits all" therapies including multiple vitamins, nutritional diets, and detoxification for unproven toxins.

The hope of this book is that parents will be better consumers to question the validity and outcome measures of such biased practice techniques. These practices may have hurt more than promoted the advancement of medicine to help in ASD. Yet this has not stopped occasional newspaper reports of mothers observing their child has improved despite no clear medical evidence documenting improvement. Usually these news reports are press releases from the various agencies promoting these alternative groups, which newspapers run without critical review because of need for a story on autism that week. These types of media stories do not prove the effectiveness of alternative treatment center programs. It is important in the face of the crisis of having an autistic child that parents remain grounded and not accept at face value the testimonials of these types of practitioners and the hype they sell. Even if some of these practitioners have good intentions, they are often misled themselves. Parents must arm themselves to ask appropriate questions and be skeptical of anyone offering to cure autism, or actively marketing themselves as autism specialists.

Chapter 17

Non-Medically Sanctioned Alternative Approaches

In my experience, there are often fringe groups promoting theories with no basis in research and facilitating laboratory testing from less respected sources or a handful of alternative laboratories. Leading examples are the varying self-promoting groups dedicated to treating autism with multi-vitamin protocols, diets, and chelation, or the nutritional-based approaches only without any neurological approach to the child. There are no specific requirements to be such a practitioner. There are also other clinics which profess knowledge of nutritional, metal, or vitamin deficiency as a root of all diseases, now including autistic spectrum disorders (ASD), but also bipolar, chronic fatigue syndrome and fibromyalgia among other chronic ailments. Interestingly, no standard laboratory studies, electroencephalography (EEG), or neuroimaging is part of this process. Often these recommendations are from physicians or biochemists not trained specifically in child development, neurology, or psychiatry. The firms and specialty laboratories used by such doctors are not specifically accredited, nor do they have control values for normal children truly to make sense of the testing done. Groups of non-useful tests that are done may confuse parents about what really is the biological basis of autism. These tests are often very costly and often not paid for by insurance, therefore increasing even more wastefully the financial burden to affected families.

Rather than mention specific names of these laboratories or firms, I will describe my professional opinion as a board-certified child neurologist on the lack of scientific value of these laboratory tests.

The most frequent abuse is hair analysis. A very good paper from the American Medical Association journal *JAMA* showed that the top three hair analysis laboratories in the United States gave different results on the same hair samples sent to each laboratory at the same time, showing lack of validity. These tests are supposed to help determine exposure to toxins, yet are influenced by diet, rate of hair growth, chemicals in pool water or shampoos, as well as the sources of local drinking water. These are not clinically very reliable for any metal toxin exposure. The main use is in cases of obvious acute poisoning, such as arsenic.

Urine tests are used for metal toxicity, specifically mercury. There are no clinically useful tests for urine screening for mercury poisoning unless tested within 24 hours of toxic mercury exposure, not remote poisoning years or months ago. Chelating agents that are used to induce excretion of metal or toxins in post-chelation urine samples do not confirm or guide treatment for theoretical increased mercury levels. Although there have been reports by one Defeat Autism Now practitioner in 2003 citing increased urinary mercury excretion, this has not been duplicated and the more recent findings of the CHARGE study at the MIND Institute has found no increased levels of mercury burden in patients with autism vs. controls. In my practice experience I have seen no conclusive proof linking body burden of mercury to patients with autism.

Yeast metabolites in urine are another mythology promoted by one laboratory. Random urine samples sent to one of these laboratories during a research study with antibiotics in autism showed no difference in defining yeast or bacterial metabolites between controls and treatment groups. Stool samples are often requested as part of these alternative treatment work-ups. Yeast in aerobic non-refrigerated stool samples or stool dysbiosis labeling have no real diagnostic value. Exposing stool samples to the air during sample collection kills the majority of stool bacteria called anaerobes. In unrefrigerated and non-anaerobic conditions, bacterial and yeast overgrowth occurs as the competing anaerobes are dead. Therefore these samples do not reflect the true nature of what is really happening in the guts of autistic children.

Certain IgG food screening tests using blood testing are of no value as many people can still eat food even if IgG antibodies to those foods exist. For instance, one patient's mother told me her son's autism was screened by a chiropractor with such tests and she was told he was allergic to shellfish, pineapple and papaya. However, when asked if he ever ate any of these when he regressed or even currently, the answer was of course "No."

Also milk and dairy products are now in the scope of blame among the lay literature of ASD. If milk allergy is suspected, go to a board-certified pediatric gastroenterologist or allergist, rather than the self-proclaimed "expert in autism" practices around the country today. There is evidence of lactose intolerance as well in autism, perhaps as high as 40 to 50 percent, so a trial of lactose tablets or lactose-free products can always be done. However, a gastroenterologist or medical allergist can be consulted to confirm these issues. Lactose intolerance is different than a milk allergy.

Wheat allergies or gluten foods have also been incriminated by the lay public as a cause of autism. Interestingly, there is some medical evidence of a loose association of celiac disease and neurological conditions in adults. Certain rare cases of brain calcifications on brain computerized axiol tomography (CAT) scans have been observed in some wheat-sensitive families from the Indian subcontinent. Northern Europeans sensitive to gluten have severe gastrointestinal problems, but milder cases can be difficult to diagnose. There are standardized medical tests which should be performed on children with chronic diarrhea, or failure to thrive, that can support the diagnosis of celiac sprue or gluten enteropathy of the intestines. These are the anti-gliadin antibodies of IgG and IgA types, tissue transglutamase tests (TTG), and the antiendomesial antibody tests. These are positive only if both IgA titers are elevated and anti-endomesial and even better TTG antibodies are positive. Elevated IgG levels are non-specific and unfortunately are what I have seen when a patient reports they have antibodies against gluten. I suspect these are more a non-specific marker for an overly sensitive or dysfunctional immune system and are actually cross-reacting non-specifically with something else. Often these children do not show other allergic testing to wheat or milk products. Because wheat is evolutionarily a more modern food, there may be primitive tendencies to have an allergic property towards wheat for some people.

I have in my experience had patients who had true celiac disease and autism. Treatment of their intestinal disease, which was biopsy and laboratory confirmed, led to improved gastrointestinal function and health. I am sad to report that other than less stomach discomfort and improved digestion, the other symptoms of autism were not helped by a gluten-free diet. Theories of neurotoxins from gluten or opioid-like substances are not confirmed in the medical literature. Therefore common sense is recommended. If parents do try the gluten/casein-free diet, care must be taken to balance the child's diet nutritionally. Some parents do report improved hyperactivity or less aggressive behavior on these diets, but I have never observed a resolution of ASD in any patient who came to me on these diets. Also, if the patients on this type of diet suffered from epilepsy or abnormal EEG, in my experience there was never any significant improvement while on the gluten/casein-free diet to these conditions or EEG patterns. I would say some parents report some slight improvement in hyperactivity, but this is also reported on other lower carbohydrate diets, such as the ketogenic diet. Other than these subjective reports, there has been no significant change in the child's language or functioning overall. As a neurologist who has seen other diets such as the ketogenic diet and Atkins diet for epilepsy, there are similar unsubstantiated claims of improved behavior and hyperactivity with these diets. There is one case in Greece where a child had occipital spikes on her EEG, intractable seizures and was found to have intestinal celiac disease. This patient did have her epilepsy go away after eight months on the gluten/casein-free diet.

Again, in my experience it could be a lower carbohydrate issue, or just parental involvement in the child's care and observation to maintain the diet that may lead to better behavior. Despite my experience that the gluten/casein-free diet does not have a major effect on ASD, medically if a parent wants to try the diet and does so under good nutritional supervision, there is no harm. Several medical centers are doing controlled testing and researching to see if there is a true improvement in ASD with this type of diet, so in the future a more scientific answer will be available to parents and physicians regarding this dietary intervention.

There are claims made by certain alternative treatment clinics where only vitamin therapy is offered or metalloprotein deficiency is diagnosed. This conclusion is made by ratios of copper or zinc being claimed as abnormal, yet the standard laboratory values are normal. There are numerous metalloproteins in all human brains and not just one simple type. Zinc and copper have both positive and potentially toxic effects. There are no simple formulas or scientific outcome studies to support supplementation with these agents, and at the same time, chelating metals from the body, as is the common practice at least one center I am aware of in the Chicago region. This can be potentially dangerous. This again seems illogical and has no scientific proof of working. There are no controlled or even clinical outcome studies of open label trials that show a positive behavioral improvement with these treatments. In my experience as a child neurologist, I have never seen a substantial benefit from chelation therapies in ASD. Again, the National Institute of Health in the United States will be doing a controlled chelation study sometime in the near future, which I hope will put this issue in a clearer perspective.

Allergies cannot be detected from holding onto a light or thermocoupled devices often used by chiropractors, naturopaths, or other non-medical practitioners. As mentioned before, immunoassays of allergic screening to multiple foods by IgG techniques is not adequate proof of food allergies.

Interpreting scientific findings

Medical scientists require research and observations to be proven with scientific and controlled methods. Sometimes pilot studies just offer observations of treatment outcome. Placebo effect is very high in ASD treatments, especially in non-controlled studies without placebo vs. treatment. Basing outcomes of treatments on phone surveys of parents and testimonials are the only evidence offered when standard medicine has asked these alternative practitioners to prove their claims of efficacy. This is often based on voluntary questionnaires filled out by self-referred parents. There are no controls for exact dosing, time given, of other variables with this data collecting technique. Parents basically answer if the child got better, got worse, or there was no effect. Now when these parents reported on various alternative or vitamin therapies, the ratios of better/worse seem to get much higher especially with certain vitamins, such as vitamin A and B6, magnesium, chelation, and digestive enzymes, sometimes having ratios of better/worse of 14–27: 1. At first this appears much better than standard drugs. However, there is another column which is "no difference" which averages between 40 to 60 percent for both vitamin and pharmaceutical drug therapies. The ratios are higher and give a false impression of more people getting better because there were fewer negative reports of side-effects with vitamins than drugs. If looking at the ratio of "no difference/better" from chelation, vitamin A, B6, magnesium, or secretin, the ratios were 1:1 or no real effect. This is because roughly 50 percent reported no change vs. less than or equal to 50 percent reporting improvement. Therefore great caution in interpreting this type of data must be exercised by parents or physicians looking at these claims from alternative groups promoting certain therapies based on such testimonial responses analyzing alternative treatment effects in ASD.

Conclusion

Most physicians like me truly want a cure or an effective treatment for many of the symptoms of autism. Please do not believe that standard medicine does not want to use holistic or vitamin therapy because of our egos. If things work and truly help the health of children with ASD, then I and most of my colleagues will use those treatments. I caution parents to use the same common sense they use for television infomercials and weight loss advertisements and not blindly follow therapies that offer instant hope but no proof of working. This is especially true for some clinics or alternative practitioners who charge large fees for unnecessary testing procedures and selling of treatments or products to help. Do not be seduced by what I call treatment "du jour."

In later chapters when treatments of ASD are discussed, more specific discussion of alternative therapies and the presence or lack of scientific evidence on treatment effectiveness will be reviewed. The next step is how to get the right type of help with the medical treatment of ASD.

Chapter 18

Overview of Medicines
No Cure, but Symptomatic Treatments Can Help

The prior chapters have been building a case that medical knowledge concerning some basic scientific facts in autistic spectrum disorders (ASD) is increasing. In addition, some limited studies of different drugs that affect behavior in ASD have been published. The case was also made that ASD is a spectrum disorder. Different problems exist for different subgroups clinically, and any treatments will not be "one size fits all." Therefore, medicines will be discussed based in clinical presentations of autistic and ASD types of children. These will be broken down by clinical presentation types. Also, I again emphasize that there are no medical consensus groups proposing a standardized treatment for ASD at this time. No parts of this book are a prescription for care, nor is this book to be used as a diagnostic or medical treatment plan. I am absolutely not recommending any specific treatment to any reader of this book. I am merely trying to explain what is known and currently has some evidence of helping. Possible future treatments may be occasionally discussed. The reader can use this book to work with a physician to open a logical dialogue for discussing medical treatments that may alleviate symptoms and improve function and quality of life for patients with ASD.

Clinical differences in subtypes of ASD
Before discussing treatment choices, it is my clinical experience that different clinical subtypes respond to different clinical treatments. There are both

primary symptoms of autism, and secondary complications including dysfunctional immune problems, abnormal electroencephalograms (EEG), sleep problems, and eating or gastrointestinal dysfunction. Any subtype of ASD may have some or all of these secondary problems.

The main categories of special subtypes that I will discuss will be: autism without language production delay; autism with expressive language delay; autism with receptive and expressive language delay (patients in this group may be more likely to have an abnormal EEG in my clinical experience); Asperger's patients, and patients in all subtypes with manic or childhood bipolar behavior. By definition core symptoms of autism or pervasive developmental disorders (PDD) have language and social delays, so these will overlap all subtypes. Also sleep problems, gastrointestinal problems, and immune problems may overlap all subtypes. Hyperactivity or attention problems affect many groups including Asperger's syndrome. Some medicines work better in some clinical presentations than others. It is assumed that patients with known genetic or metabolic disorders that mimic ASD are not included in this discussion. The following recommendations will be for ASD from idiopathic or unknown causes.

Autism subtypes without language production delay

The types of patients in this category may produce speech sounds and have sentences but use language in rigid or stereotypic manners. This group usually will have normal EEG, will not have clinically regressed, and may be diagnosed later as having a problem. Usually functional intellect is in the low normal or normal range. This group is referred to as high-functioning autism. Also in this class are the Asperger's subtypes. This group usually does not have sleep disorders. They may have anxiety or obsessive traits, and this group often has trouble with attention deficit symptoms. There can be some aggression but less than in lower-functioning groups, and when it occurs may be from a panic or anxiety trigger in my experience. Some degree of auditory processing dysfunction may exist. Frontal lobe tasks for executive function and multitasking is impaired to varying degrees in this group.

The medications that may play a role here may be medications for attention deficit disorder, such as stimulants or non-stimulants. For the anxiety and obsessional behaviors sometimes anti-anxiety medications in the form of serotonin reuptake inhibitors (SSRIs) can be useful. If delusional or overly compulsive traits are present, sometimes atypical antipsychotic medications are useful. For executive functioning the frontal lobe medications that are also used in Alzheimer's disease may be helpful; these include cholinesterase inhibitors and glutamine blockers like memantine. Also L-carnosine may help auditory processing.

Autism subtypes with language apraxia/no receptive language-processing delay

These patients may have intelligence quotient (IQ) testing levels of 40 to 80 and often appear to be lower functioning. This group of children usually never had functional language, due to frontal lobe dysfunction and oral motor apraxia. They usually have oral motor feeding problems. The magnetic resonance imaging (MRI) studies on this group are usually normal, and no defects in the brain structure are visible despite obvious malfunction of the oral motor region. If this group has normal or near normal receptive language, then the main goal of medical therapy is to get these children to try to talk. Although oral motor therapy is helpful, the speech apraxia (lack of motor skills in tongue and mouth muscles to initiate speech) is usually refractive. This suggests a brain dysfunction in the prefrontal and opercular regions of the brain, specifically the dominant hemisphere (left usually).

These patients do not have a specific medication that helps their oral motor planning. There have rarely been some responses in some children to memantine (an Alzheimer's medication that blocks glutamine and N-methyl D aspartate (NMDA) receptors), but no real response to cholinesterase inhibitors. For frustration and behaviors, atypical antipsychotics may be useful in lower-functioning children. Alternative communication devices called augmentative communication devices like the Picture Exchange Communication System (PECS) or voice box technology may be helpful. The group of pure isolated oral motor dysfunction in ASD is small, as there are other associated fine motor and receptive speech problems in the majority of these patients.

Autism subtypes with receptive language deficits with or without regression

These children are of two types: Children always delayed in receptive language from infancy onward and those that develop some initial early speech but then regress and seem to become less responsive to spoken language between 15 and 24 months of age. Sometimes parents fear the latter type may seem to become deaf to speech. Early self-stimulatory behaviors may be absent and develop between 24 and 36 months. Rarely there is more than one regression. The regression may be rapid or slow and insidious. Both of these types may have a higher risk of abnormal EEG, especially, as mentioned, with an overnight study.

These groups, especially with the apparent regression, may respond to a variety of medications for their receptive speech deficits. If the EEG is abnormal, my experience has been best in roughly 70 percent using valproic acid medication. If the EEG is abnormal and there is regression or clear associated risk factors or family history of immune dysfunction, then corticosteroids may also reverse the auditory receptive processing delays. With normalized or always normal EEG groups, medications that further enhance receptive language include the cholinesterases; memantine is especially good, and L-carnosine as a non-prescription supplement. These children may rarely benefit from these with increased oral motor function efforts as well. Expected gains could be better enunciation or increased length of utterances. Oral motor function is harder to stimulate than the receptive function. Supportive speech therapy is useful, especially combined with medications. Patients with a history of no expressive language usually fare worse in levels of speech recovery expressively. Behavioral aggression and attention may also need to be addressed in this group.

Asperger's syndrome

This group usually starts with fluent verbal language but may have attention and anxiety and obsessive-compulsive traits. The Asperger's group tends to have less frequently abnormal EEG tracings. Also they respond better to stimulants for their attention than more typical autistics. SSRI medications also respond better in this group in general. Spelling and phonic issues may be more likely in this group. They are less bothered in general than high-functioning autistics by environmental background noise. This group is less likely to have sleep dysfunction and are less likely to have epilepsy or abnormal EEG patterns. High normal or above IQ levels are found typically.

Manic or childhood bipolar types

This behavioral pattern seen in many patients with ASD overlaps all of the above subtypes. There can be normal or abnormal language, regression or none, high or low functioning. This group often has atypical hyperactive behavior, may react negatively to stimulants or SSRIs. This group may have rapid mood changes going from laughing to crying. They may draw or play with certain toys in an endless fashion. They may play with many different things at once.

Often these children are poor sleepers, especially at maintaining sleep. They can often be highly irritable infants. They may talk excessively about topics like movies. They can become easily agitated for no reason.

These children respond to mood stabilizing anti-epileptic drugs like valproic acid, lithium, and atypical antipsychotics. Any of the above subtypes can be affected in this way. Family history of bipolar conditions or atypical schizophrenia may help make this diagnosis more likely as well.

Clinical problems across subtypes

Gastrointestinal reflux or constipation symptoms

Any subtype can have trouble with gastroesophageal reflux; in fact there may be up to 40 to 50 percent suffering from this with ASD. This is often missed by lack of pain response or lack of communication in these children. Sudden changes in appetite, irritability relieved by constant eating, making themselves vomit, and hitting of chest may be heartburn- or reflux-related. These are treated with antacids, histamine H2 receptor blocking agents, and sometimes dietary treatment. Lactose intolerance can be treated by diet and lactase enzyme tablets. If combining drugs for reflux, make sure how they interact with the absorption of other drugs being used.

Constipation or constipation alternating with diarrhea is common in ASD as well. This is again a comorbidity for any subtype above. Colonic decompression by enemas and chronic laxative therapy is often needed. Secretin (a pancreatic hormone), although touted as being beneficial in ASD, has not been shown to improve any of the core symptoms. It may even worsen some subtypes of ASD causing tics and worse behaviors.

Sleep problems

Sleep disorders are common in ASD. There can be typical childhood sleep apnea due to adenoid or tonsilar abnormalities, restless legs, sleep onset disorders, or waking in the middle of the night with insomnia. Some children have combined types of sleep dysfunction. Sleep disruption may be seen in 50 percent or more of ASD patients.

For sleep onset problems, induction of sleep by routine and structure may help, but often medications are needed. Good effects have been obtained with melatonin, alpha-adrenergic blockers like tizanidine or clonidine, and occasionally other medications. Benzodiazepines often agitate or have the opposite effects.

Sleep maintenance problems should be examined by overnight EEG and polysomnogram studies where indicated. Decreased REM (rapid eye movement) sleep may be present especially in the manic group. Mood stabilizers like valproic acid or other drugs that affect sleep cycles like antidepressants and other anticonvulsants may be helpful. If restless legs syndrome is found, then supplements for iron deficiency, or certain treatments for dopaminergic deficiency, may be helpful. If the EEG is abnormal, then anti-epileptic drugs like valproic acid are very useful in sleep maintenance. Last, gastric reflux or abdominal pain may disrupt sleep in some children with ASD.

Immune problems

If recurrent infection and proven immunoglobulin deficiency is present, some patients may have a concurrent mild immune deficiency. Some treat this on a selected case-by-case basis with intravenous immunoglobulins (IVIG). If autoimmune regression is suspected, the most likely treatment has been a form of corticosteroid. Again, these treatments are to be used in the rare case of ASD only when clinical evidence supports the risks or the costs of this type of therapy.

Summary

The following chapters will focus more specifically on classes of medications used in ASD. More details of treatment will be discussed. Judiciously used, medications can improve the quality of life for the patient and family in a number of ways. Improved sleep helps the entire family function better. Decreased irritability or self-injury is obviously a benefit. Treatment of receptive speech delay by treating an abnormal EEG or trying the medications that have been shown to improve receptive language can greatly enhance the function and communication of a child with ASD. Improved gastrointestinal and sleep function help the day-to-day behavior in these children, Each child with ASD is a different subtype potentially and no single treatment may apply to every case. Always be cautious of promises of cures and "cookie cutter" approaches that offer the same treatment for everyone with ASD.

PART V

Neurologically Managing Clinical Aspects with Medication

Chapter 19

Medicines Prescribed for Behavioral Problems

Medications used in autistic spectrum disorders (ASD) are chosen by experienced physicians to treat various symptoms associated with ASD. There are subtypes of ASD and therefore a variety of different clinical behavioral problems that do not all respond in some "cookie cutter" fashion to the same treatments. There are currently no cures for ASD. Drugs that give symptomatic relief are of various categories. They address symptoms such as aggression, movement disorders like tics, self-injury, and obsessive behaviors. There are antidepressants and anti-anxiety medications. There are also subtypes of ASD with bipolar-type mood swings, aggression, or mania. Antipsychotic or mood-stabilizing medications are useful in that group. Hyperactivity and attention problems also are often present with ASD.

Subsequent chapters will deal with other medication options in ASD. There is some experimental evidence that certain drugs improve electroencephalograms (EEG) or behavior, and these also treat seizures in ASD. There are medications experimentally used for the immune system or disordered thinking in ASD. There are medications for gastrointestinal problems or sleep disruption. Currently, none of these medications are FDA (Food and Drug Administration in the United States) approved for ASD-specific treatment. In addition, some are not even yet officially approved for use in children, even though many pediatric specialists do use them with child patients. Parents need the guidance of an experienced physician to help make decisions as to their own individual safety and comfort level for the medications discussed in this book as being useful in ASD. I must emphasize again that this book is for educational use only and should not be used as recommending any particular therapy. Only in consultation with a trained specialist dealing with pediatric or adult cases of ASD should medical treatment decisions be made. For the clarity of these chapters I will mostly use brand names more recognizable for parents.

Antipsychotics: Dopamine-blocking agents

The term antipsychotic is a very misleading term for this group of medications. There is currently no professional that believes that the ASD are disorders of infantile psychosis or childhood schizophrenia, although in the past this was contemplated. Actually the role of these agents is to inhibit certain dopamine receptors which may, when excessively stimulated, cause manic or delusional behavior. Overt aggression, self-picking or mutilation, and various tic movements are treated with these medications. In child psychiatry and neurology these medications are used for a variety of disorders. Most typically they are used for Tourette's syndrome, aggressive or violent behavior, acute or chronic forms of manic depression, and sometimes atypical attention deficit disorder and hyperactivity.

These agents comprise a new and older group. The older group affects mainly the D2 dopamine receptor. These can have hypothalamic effects that can elevate the hormone prolactin. These older agents can cause excessive weight gain through increased appetite. Also they can cause a form of Parkinson's type movements, such as cogwheeling or dystonic type reactions that are reversible and treatable. The older drugs can also rarely cause a severe involuntary movement disorder called tardive dyskinesia due to dopamine receptor dysfunction. This unfortunately can be paradoxical, unpredictable, and often permanent and irreversible. Luckily it is rare, but for this reason these drugs are not first choice among the dopamine-blocking agents.

The most common commercial drugs of this type are Haldol (haloperidol), Thorazine (chlorpromazine), and Mellaril (thioridazine). These do less for anxiety, depression, or obsessive conditions than newer agents. For tics, Haldol and a less risky drug Orap may still be preferred, and sometimes these older drugs are better for self-injury and aggression in severe cases.

Newer agents began with Risperdal (risperidone) and Clozaril (clozapine). These also affect D2 receptors, but also D3 and D5 receptors. These drugs can also have some effect on the serotonin receptors more like an antidepressant.

These agents block some receptors, but also stimulate others. Clozaril can be dangerous and, rarely, has caused bone marrow failure. It is very effective, but frequent blood tests that are required make it hard to use in ASD, only when all other drugs fail. It is not used in children usually because of the risk of bone marrow failure and required weekly blood tests for the first six months, followed then by tests every other week. This vigilant monitoring is not the case for the other agents.

Risperdal (risperidone) is the only drug tested in a well-controlled large autism study by the RUPP (Research Units for Pediatric Psychiatry) groups at multi-center research sites. This testing and vast experience has even finally led to FDA approval in 2007 for the treatment of symptoms related to autism in children over age five years. This is the first such approved drug in the United States. Prior open label studies with Haldol and Mellaril were not well controlled. Risperdal is used in Tourette's as well. Risperdal still causes side-effects of weight gain and can cause elevated prolactin levels and sedation. Rarely, a benign tumor called a hypothalamic adenoma may occur in approximately 1:240,000 patients. Newer agents are related to Risperdal and include Zyprexa (olazepine), Geodon (ziprasidone), Seroquel (quetiapine), and Abilify (aripiprazole). Most of these are not well tested in pediatrics, but all have been used by some physicians for ASD. They are not FDA-approved for ASD, and many are not yet approved for pediatric use by the FDA. Therefore drug manufacturers cannot promote pediatric use at this time. Despite this, a physician may have good reasons to try some of these agents in a given patient.

Most common side effects of the newer atypical antipsychotic class of medications are fatigue, nausea, dizziness, sedation, and weight gain from increased appetite. Dangers from these medications include excessive weight gain that can lead to what is called "metabolic syndrome" which is a pre-diabetic condition similar to adult-onset type 2 diabetes. These children may have elevated prolactin hormone levels, except for those treated with Seroquel and Abilify. This may lead to increased breast tissue and, rarely, lactation. Rare chances for a benign pituitary brain tumor called an adenoma have been reported, the highest incidences with Haldol and Risperdal (1:240,000 cases). Again, despite these risks, for the majority these drugs are statistically safe. Decisions to use these drugs are only to be made by an experienced physician. They should be used for symptoms of aggression, self-abuse, and manic subtypes of ASD. They can lower seizure resistance thresholds as well in ASD children with epilepsy. Therefore caution is needed in adding these medications to patients with abnormal EEG or clinical seizures histories. See Table 19.1 for a summary.

Table 19.1 Summary of antipsychotic medications used in ASD

Antipsychotic medications	Prior reported medical use in ASD	FDA-approved for children or ASD	High risk dystonia or tardive dyskinesia	Risk of weight gain
Haldol	YES	YES, not ASD	YES +++	+++
Mellaril	YES	NO	YES +++	+++
Risperdal	YES	YES, YES ASD	YES +	+++
Zyprexa	YES	NO	YES +	++++
Seroquel	YES	NO	NO +/_	++
Geodon	YES	NO	NO +/_	+
Abilify	YES	NO	NO	+/_

Key: +/_ = none or equivocal; + = low; ++ = medium; +++ = high; ++++ = very high

Antidepressant medications

There are many patients with ASD who suffer from anxiety, or have severe compulsive or obsessive behaviors. Sometimes the stress and realization that they are different leads patients actually to become depressed with acting out and aggressive outbursts. It is often difficult to tell from the history whether aggression is random or the result of anxiety or depression in a child or adult with ASD. Often it is necessary to question the caregiver about what leads to or provokes the unwanted behaviors. What is from situational anxiety versus random acting out? Does the child realize what they are doing or do they seem in their own world? These details help the physician to select a medication appropriately. For instance, when a child acts out from a fantasy world or manic state, they may need an antipsychotic medication instead of an antidepressant. However, if the acting out is from performance or transitional anxiety then the choice of an antidepressant may be helpful. This section will focus on the tricyclic and SSRI (selective serotonin reuptake inhibitors) types of antidepressants.

Antidepressants have been available for the past 30 years, and early tricyclic types (named for shape of molecular structure) were helpful for increasing norepinephrine levels. They were sedating, and still may help with sleep-onset problems. They did not address severe anxiety well, nor did they address obsessive-compulsive disorder (OCD) issues. These medications sometimes address atypical attention issues. They can agitate or worsen bipolar type conditions. These drugs, especially Elavil (amitriptyline), Norpramine (desipramine), and Tofranil (imipramine), have sedating properties and pain properties. They are used in headache and sleep-onset disorders at times. They can cause constipation and dry mouth as a result of anti-cholinergic action. This may be cognitively detrimental in ASD conditions. These drugs are rarely used today as first line agents, but sometimes for sleep induction or maintenance.

The first drug for OCD was related to the tricyclics and named Anafranil. This drug has some use in severe OCD and has been somewhat useful in ASD. This medication has really been replaced by the SSRI class of medications. The SSRI medications are familiar as Prozac (fluoxetine), Zoloft (sertraline), Celexa (citralopram), Luvox (fluvoxamine), Paxil (paroxetine), and Lexapro (escitalopram). These medications block the local reuptake of serotonin after release between neuronal junctions, effectively increasing available serotonin. These drugs work well for social or situational panic or anxiety, and also for obsessive-compulsive type behaviors. These often do not help self-mutilation such as picking skin scabs or hair pulling in the ASD population because these behaviors are often more related to tics than OCD. These may therefore respond better to the dopamine-blocking agents.

Another similar class of drugs useful and similar to the SSRI drugs is the mixed class of agents that work on both some serotonin and norepinephrine effect. These may help anxiety, and some symptoms of OCD. These agents may still induce manic reactions in patients, but may have less overt serotonin effects. These drugs are Effexor (venlafaxine), Cymbalta (duloxetine), and Wellbutrin (bupropion). Some of these drugs may help attention more than pure SSRI agents due to the norepinephrine effect that pure SSRI agents lack. Therefore these drugs may work for some patients as well as SSRI medications for anxiety, but may also have some positive effect on attention through the norepenephrine effect.

The important message for all antidepressants in the ASD population is that these drugs, by increasing available serotonin and norepinephrine, may trigger agitated or manic states in patients who may have underlying bipolar conditions as part of ASD. Often these drugs are best used in very small amounts in the ASD population. They are often more useful in the Asperger's subtypes. The doses may range from a tenth to a quarter of an adult dose of SSRI upon initiation, and titration should be carefully monitored by your physician. A summary of these antidepressants is available in Table 19.2.

Table 19.2 Summary of antidepressant medications used in ASD

Antidepressant medications	Classification	Studies published in ASD	Side-effects	Formulation
Elavil	Tricyclics: (Norepinephrine Selective)	Rarely	Dry mouth	Liquid/tablet
Pamelor	Tricyclics: (Norepinephrine Selective)	No	Constipation	Tablet
Desipramine	Tricyclics: (Norepinephrine Selective)	No	Weight gain, sedation	Tablet
Anafranil	Tricyclic Variant (Serotonin Selective)	Yes	Sedation, weight gain	Capsule
Prozac	SSRI	Yes	Mania/hyperactivity, insomnia	Capsule/tablet/liquid
Effexor	SSRI/NERI	Yes	Mania	Capsule
Cymbalta	SSRI/NERI	No	Mania	Tablet
Paxil	SSRI	Yes	Sedation, activation/mania, weight gain	Tablet/liquid
Zoloft	SSRI	Yes	Similar to Prozac	Tablet/liquid
Luvox	SSRI	Yes	Similar to Prozac	Tablet
Celexa/Lexapro	SSRI	Yes	Similar to Prozac	Tablet/liquid

In summary the antidepressants are useful for irritable or anxious behavior in some children with ASD. Although there is some evidence on positron emission tomography (PET) scans that serotonin metabolism may be abnormal, these serotonergic drugs have been disappointing with their limited effectiveness overall. There may be some patients with serotonin transporter gene defects of ASD that may respond better than others to these drugs; however, this will be a subject of future research as these genes are just recently discovered and not clinically being utilized in planning specific treatment yet. The SSRI medications are the most widely used of the antidepressants. The older agents, with the exception of Anafranil, are rarely used today. Elavil is the most likely one; it is used for headaches and to help initiate sleep in this population.

Medications for hyperactivity and inattention

There are many children with ASD that appear to be inattentive and suffer from some symptoms of hyperactivity. Despite these clinical appearances, the response to stimulants and other medications for hyperactivity or attention deficit disorder (ADD/ADHD) has been less than desired in the majority of experiences. Often children with ASD respond negatively to stimulant medications. This section will focus on the medications used for these types of behaviors and where these medications may be effective.

Stimulants and non-stimulants

Medical strategies used for typically developing children with ADD or ADHD are based predominantly on the stimulant class of medications. These products include Ritalin regular and long acting, or derivatives using the generic form methylphenidate, Concerta, Metadate, and Methylin and other brands in the United States. Products using the right-sided isomer of Ritalin are called Focalin. The other major stimulant group consists of dextroamphetamine salt derivatives Dexedrine, Adderall products, and other less used amphetamines. The Ritalin-derived drugs increase dopamine to the frontal region and cingulate gyrus of the cerebral cortex, while the amphetamine-based derivatives work to increase both dopamine and norepinephrine levels. The elevation of these chemical neurotransmitters may cause the adverse manic or overly agitated behaviors seen in many ASD children who adversely respond to stimulants.

Although in typically developing children, the ADD/ADHD response is usually dramatically positive with decreased hyperactivity and better attention in 75 to 80 percent of those treated, in ASD patients there has been disappointment in the response in clinical studies that have looked at these issues. The RUPP group and others have only formally studied immediate release methylphenidate (Ritalin), and none of the other stimulants to date have been systematically studied. Although there can be a 30 to 50 percent rate of hyperactive or attention improvement, 50 to 70 percent of the patients may develop adverse side-effects when typical autism or pervasive developmental disorder (PDD) is also present. One observation is that the Asperger's group tolerates stimulants better than other ASD subtypes. Also adverse events that occur more often in ASD than in typical ADHD children are agitation, irritability, increased over-focused or self-stimulatory behaviors, while this population still experiences the increased tics, insomnia, and decreased appetite seen in typically developed children with ADD or ADHD. The main purpose of trying these stimulant agents is that they are short-acting, have a rapid response, and within one or two days a change in treatment strategy can be done if the medication does not work or has too much of an adverse effect. The general advice is that children over eight years of age with ADHD symptoms and ASD respond better than younger patients, and Asperger's type patients may tolerate stimulants better than other subtypes of the ASD spectrum. Also a negative response to a stimulant in a manic or hyperactive child with ASD may guide the treating physician to consider whether a bipolar subtype may be present in that patient. This negative response may help guide a change to a different treatment pathway.

The non-stimulant medication Strattera (atomoxetine), which is a norepinephrine reuptake inhibitor (NERI), and some tricyclic antidepressants work to increase norepinephrine. This is modeled after the SSRI mechanism seen in the antidepressant section. These have not yet been well studied in ASD. Strattera does little for the hyperactive groups, but may help some inattentive types of ADD children. However, there are no formal studies yet in ASD. Personal experience is that Strattera may help some school-age children with ASD, but still can exacerbate mania and does carry this as a prescription warning in typically developing children. Older antidepressants and some newer agents are used in some cases where stimulants and Strattera have failed. These include Tofranil, Desipramine, Wellbutrin, Effexor, among others. These have limited usefulness in ASD in selected cases.

Another class agent is Provigil (generic modafinil, trade name for ADD yet unknown) which was previously used in narcolepsy. This non-specifically stimulates the frontal lobe. Although not supposedly acting through dopaminergic pathways, in my clinical experience this agent has acted similar to stimulants and caused activation and mania in the ASD patients in general experience in my clinical use. There are no formal studies yet. This agent will probably have limited use in ASD with hyperactive symptoms.

Alpha agonists and antipsychotics

The children who respond poorly to stimulants or are aggressive may respond better to alpha agonists that block norepinephrine responses that may cause aggression. These medications include Catapress (clonidine), Tenex (guanfacine), and Zanaflex (tizanidine). These drugs are also used in childhood tic disorders, and Tourette's syndrome. They are used for impulsive aggression, and may help some hyperactivity, but have limited effect on attention. These drugs may be sedating, and are often used for sleep-onset aid in children with ADHD or ASD. Limited studies in autism have shown help with impulsivity. Again higher-functioning or Asperger's subtypes may respond better.

Antipsychotics as mentioned above for aggression probably help by blocking dopamine receptors and helping out in cases of manic or bipolar subtypes of ASD that mimic hyperactive symptoms. These medications are also used for sleep and tic disorders in some patients with ASD as well. These drugs do little directly for inattention.

Mood-stabilizing medications

In ASD, there are often symptoms that are characterized by lability of moods: often happy one minute, then crying; or excessively energetic as if powered by a motor, followed by a sudden loss of wanting to do things. These behaviors are frequent in ASD. Differentiating manic energy from hyperactivity is often a clinical guess. Sometimes a negative response to stimulants used to treat hyperactivity, or manic activation of irritability by SSRI antidepressants, gives a clue that a bipolar-type biochemistry may be present in a given patient. These patients may have either an abnormal or normal EEG. Choices of medication are helped by the knowledge of whether an abnormal EEG is present. Perhaps an anti-epileptic drug that also acts as a mood stabilizing medication may be helpful, while an antipsychotic may worsen an abnormal EEG or even lower resistance to having a clinical seizure. A baseline EEG may therefore be a very useful tool when making medication choices in this population.

Mood stabilizers help in different ways. The classic mood-stabilizing drug is lithium which works by an unknown mechanism. Side-effects are well known and can be monitored. There can be weight gain, but not as severe as the antipsychotic medicines already discussed. Lithium levels can be monitored, but there is a narrow therapeutic window that is between 0.5 to 1.8 mg/dl in the blood. Tremors, thyroid interference, and potential heart rhythm disturbances can occur with high lithium levels that are above 2.5 to 3 mg/dl. Therefore knowledge of lithium side-effects and patient compliance are important in ASD patients that require this treatment.

Anticonvulsants that have proven useful in adult or pediatric bipolar patients include Depakote/Depakene (valproic acid), Lamictal (lamotrigine), and also Tegretol/Carbatrol (carbamazepine) or Trileptol (oxcarbazepine). These are drugs that may protect against seizures. Only valproic acid and possibly to some degree lamotrigine are helpful in improving EEG abnormalities such as spike patterns. In some epileptic cognitive conditions such as Lennox-Gastaut syndrome or Landau-Kleffner syndrome, Tegretol or Trileptol may worsen spike-wave patterns on EEG. This may be negative also in the ASD patient with an abnormal generalized EEG and bipolar symptoms. Lamotrigine may help the more chronically depressed patient who has infrequent mood swings but is mostly chronically irritable, while valproic acid and lithium products seem to help more rapidly cycling mood patterns. I have found that higher valproic acid levels are useful in ASD patients, as with bipolar patients who benefit from this drug. It is my experience that levels above 90 mg/dl to 120 mg/dl may be the useful therapeutic range for valproic acid in ASD. In fact, I have observed that patients with valproic acid levels of less than 80 mg/dl as a trough or early morning level often have worse clinical behaviors, while the higher range (90 to 120 mg/dl) often has better behavioral results. If you have tried valproic acid with less than expected results, this is one factor that needs to be reviewed to make sure the drug was adequately utilized.

Self-injury and aggressive behaviors

Subpopulations with ASD, particularly lower-functioning, mentally impaired, and less verbal groups, may act out with aggression or self-injury when frustrated or angry. This is sometimes due to anxiety, or frustration with inability to communicate basic needs. Sometimes there is no obvious reason for the self-injurious behaviors observed. In rare cases this can be very severe, bordering on self-abusive or serious physical self-inflicted injury. These cases can be very difficult to manage pharmacologically. Sometimes the SSRIs help anxiety, but worsen mania and aggression; sometimes antipsychotic medications cause sedation or unwanted side-effects, yet poor behavior continues.

Some ASD patients with severe self-injury were once thought to be trying to increase endogenous opioids by the pain from the injury inducing an intrinsic neuronal response of increased enkephalins and endorphins, the brain's internal opioids. This theory is no longer in favor, but did yield efforts to treat with opioid-blocking agents such as Naltrexone with mixed results. Most studies did not find a positive outcome. In the RUPP and other studies looking at Risperdal, there were definite improvements in aggressive or irritable behavior in ASD patients. In cases of manic behavior, mood stabilizers such as anticonvulsants like Depakote, Lamictal, Tripleptol, and Tegretol have been tried, along with lithium with mixed results. Beta-blocking agents or alpha agonist medications have also been tried for self-abuse, but no single best treatment option exists for this difficult behavioral problem in ASD. In fact, sometimes aversive behavioral methods in extreme cases are necessary.

Sometimes arm boards, helmets, or other protective devices are utilized in severe self-injurious patients. In severe cases of self-injury, sources of underlying discomfort should be sought, like gastroesophageal reflux, headache, toothache, constipation, or other discomfort that may trigger a primitive-type reaction in a low-functioning patient. I have seen patients with gallbladder and reflux pain hit their chests very hard, and have had one patient pull out permanent teeth due to severe reflux disease that was undiagnosed. Headaches, like migraine attacks, have caused intermittent head banging. Unfortunately, in my experience, there has been severe self-injury where no source of discomfort was found to be triggering the events. This is a very difficult and emotionally trying problem for parents and physicians alike.

Medicating sleep dysfunction

Autism is a disorder that frequently has sleep disruption as one of the most common complaints. The serious nature of sleep disorders in this population has not been formally studied but in my clinical experience comprises a few clinical situations. There is a group where sleep is disturbed by nocturnal epileptic activity, and this will be discussed in the next chapter in detail. There are also sleep-onset problems that may be behavioral or anxiety-driven, and possibly from manic conditions in some patients. There are sleep disruption patterns that have awakenings after three or four hours of sleep with no sleep-onset resistance. There are also mixtures of sleep-onset and sleep-disruption patterns. I have not generally found high incidences of either sleep apnea of obstructive type in this population, or high frequencies of restless legs syndrome, either by the clinical histories or polysomnograms that I have performed. What I and others have found is decreased rapid eye movement (REM) activity and sometimes patterns that suggest abnormal REM sleep patterns that typically are seen in the elderly. These reports are in only a few cases so far in the medical literature, and more formal studies need to be performed for definitive sleep data in ASD. However, there are medical ways to help families get their children adequate sleep and therefore help the quality of life in these children now.

Sleep-onset disorders

Sleep-onset problems are not uncommon in many children with developmental disabilities, including ASD. Many children have trouble due to hyperactivity or poor body awareness recognizing when they are tired, and many may resist behaviorally going to bed. In rare cases, there are children with anxiety who are afraid to go to bed, or even more rarely children with nocturnal epilepsy who have expressed fear of having seizures at night. Most commonly, the clinical problem we see is getting the child with manic or hyperactive symptoms ready for bed into a routine to settle down.

In my experience, sedating drugs like valium (diazepam) and sleep medications like Ambien (zolpidem) and other sleep agents related to benzodiazepines can have an opposite effect. I also do not recommend Benedryl or chloral hydrate for these reasons, as well as because of a tolerance effect. The first thing to do is get the child into a regular routine before bedtime. This should be a gradual reduction from more active to less active routines with no stimulating television or music before bedtime. The child should try melatonin 1 to 3 mg, approximately 30 minutes before bedtime. If this fails to induce sleep, a trial of up to 6 mg of melatonin can be tried before switching to prescription medications for sleep onset. If melatonin is not enough for sleep onset, my next favorite medication is Zanaflex (tizanidine), an alpha adrenergic agent and a centrally acting muscle relaxant. This is started at 2 mg 20 to 30 minutes before bedtime and increased up to 8 mg. This lasts four hours and has no addictive properties. Older medications also used of this class are the drugs Catapress (clonidine) 0.1 mg tablets and Tenex (guanfesine) 1 mg. These are alpha antagonists. Sedation as a side-effect helps here for sleep onset. These agents are very successful as a class with few side-effects and little risk the next day. If these fail, a newer agent Rozerem, which is a melatonin receptor agonist, mimics melatonin receptor binding sites. This also may act to help sleep initiation. These drugs do not keep the patient asleep all night if there is a REM sleep disorder later in the sleep cycle or manic-depressive issues causing sleep awakening. Also these will not stop epileptic awakenings.

Mid-sleep cycle and REM cycle disturbances

Patients who regularly awaken in the middle of the night, perhaps three to five hours into sleeping, often have lack of REM sleep on their polysomnograms. In my clinical experience, these children may have abnormal EEG patterns in sleep. If they do have an abnormal EEG, then treatment with an anti-epileptic agent like valproic acid often corrects sleep patterns within a few days or weeks of initiation of therapy. Other medications that have helped in these cases have included lamotrigine and gabapentin. In cases where frequent awakening occurs, no definite epilepsy is present, and there is no evidence of obstructive sleep apnea or restless legs, medications that increase the REM sleep cycle are often helpful. These include Neurontin (gabapentin), Elavil (amitriptyline), and Desyrel (trazodone). Sometimes melatonin and Rozerem or Zanaflex may help initiate initial deeper sleep as well in combination.

If strong clinical evidence of severe daytime anxiety exists, treating daytime anxiety with an SSRI or mixed agent may alleviate nocturnal anxiety and help anxiety-induced sleep issues. In cases of bipolar or manic states, mood stabilizers or antipsychotic medications to treat the underlying disorder may stabilize the sleep patterns. This is often clinically true where cycles of sleep disruption occur in monthly or weekly patterns. Keeping good sleep diaries will help your physician guide therapeutic choices based on which medications may help the patient's sleep disturbances the best.

Behaviorally, it is important not to reward the patients getting up in the middle of the night. Do not allow the child to watch TV, socialize, crawl into the parents' bed, play with toys, or get food reinforcement for awakening. Good sleep behavioral management is important.

Polypharmacy

This book is a guide and each patient needs to be fully evaluated by his or her own physician. Usually in ASD, patients require polypharmacy for medical augmentation to behavior management. These patients are complex and biochemically have more than one issue needing help. This book is meant to make suggestions that parents and physicians can use to troubleshoot which medications may help, and when the medications do not help, then perhaps help find a reason why not.

There are patients that do not respond to a single medication for behavior. Some patients have bipolar-type behavior, with hyperactivity, and also sometimes sleep disorders. The average non-autistic bipolar pediatric patient in the United States is on three medications. Often a mood stabilizer needs to be combined with an antipsychotic or an antidepressant. There may still be a need to treat an abnormal EEG, treat anxiety or OCD, and treat a major sleep-onset problem. There is no one treatment option here. Sometimes, once moods are stabilized, a physician can go ahead and treat a comorbid condition such as ADHD or anxiety that coexists in a bipolar subtype of ASD. However, before the bipolar-type condition was treated, the hyperactive ADHD or anxiety issues, if treated, would have exacerbated the manic symptoms. This may work even when a medication failed before because the mood disorder was unrecognized. It is also important to realize that these patients are evolving, and go through normal changes as they age including hormonal changes. This is especially true with adolescent males going through puberty, sometimes getting more physically aggressive, and females showing more mood instability such as premenstrual syndrome. Parents and treating physicians must be prepared for medication adjustments as an ongoing part of treatment in patients with ASD. Also hormonal change may bring out mood or thought disorders for the first time just as in normal adolescents.

In addition, medication safety monitoring, especially in polypharmacy where more than one type of drug is needed for the bipolar subtypes, is essential for patients with ASD who often cannot communicate side-effects as readily as more verbally normal peers. It is very rare for more than one type of antipsychotic or anticonvulsant to be needed in a given patient. However, this author leaves all medication choices to your treating physician, so remember there can always be an exception to common treatment suggestions that physicians like me may recommend. Most importantly, when dealing with complex biochemical treatments in ASD, the patient's health and individual needs come first. It is also important to remember that supplements and alternative therapies are also pharmacologically active and may interfere with prescription medications. It is very important therefore to tell a treating physician what you are giving your child from other alternative therapists or health food shops so no unusual side-effects or drug interactions occur.

Chapter 20

Treating EEG Abnormalities and Epilepsy

Autism and autism spectrum disorders (ASD) comprise a spectrum of disorders. As a neurologist, I have found there have always been severely epileptic children who have survived catastrophic births or infantile spasms or Lennox-Gastaut syndrome and clinically had many autistic traits in their behavior. As a neurology fellow, I was studying Landau-Kleffner syndrome (LKS). I became involved by default with children referred to rule out this rare disorder who happened to have regressive subtypes of autism. I was the only pediatric neurologist in the epilepsy section, and therefore given the task of studying these autistic, non-classic LKS patients. Many had abnormal sleep electroencephalogram (EEG) patterns. This started my interest in studying this population.

As I read the literature, I became aware that very few EEG studies for overnight EEG had been performed on autistic children. Epilepsy, however, had been described ever since the first autism cases in the 1940s and provided the initial evidence that autism and ASD are biological and neurological, not just behaviorally based conditions. Later came the evidence that many patients may have abnormal EEG patterns or seizures throughout their lifespan. Within the past decade there is more evidence that autism is increasing in our society and that perhaps the types of cases are different than when first described by Leo Kanner more than 50 years ago. This in turn has led to increasing awareness that this is a biologically complex spectrum disorder, with multiple genetic and environmental factors. Recent evidence suggests that perhaps there may even exist immunologically derived components that play a role in the pathogenesis of ASD. This is paralleling epilepsy research, where inflammation is currently being studied as a trigger for evolving epileptic patterns in clinical models.

I have published data from a very large series of patients screened with overnight ambulatory EEG with initial screening for ASD. Over 60 percent of the patients had some sleep-activated epileptiform abnormalities on their overnight EEG tracings during their stages 2 and 3 of sleep. Other authors have found high frequencies of EEG abnormalities in sleep as well, ranging from 30 to 60 percent, depending on a clinical history of prior seizures and the length of EEG sampling, among other variables. Clinical seizures in this population vary in frequency from 10 to 30 percent over the lifespan. More details have already been reviewed in Chapter 8.

This chapter is not going to answer all the skeptics who argue that the EEG abnormalities are not worth treating in ASD, and it is not supposed to be just a platform for my biased opinion as an author either. I hope to present the clinical evidence of the past 15 years of my practice taking care of children with ASD and abnormal EEG patterns. I also will present what I think are intriguing arguments for early treatment of the EEG as potentially helpful for cognition, behavior, and language, even in the absence of clinical epilepsy. I also will discuss the potential risks of treatment and the need for more research. The epileptic patterns in these children may be more of an epiphenomenon than a true cause and effect, reflecting yet one more layer of dysfunction upon the autistic brain. The observations of my clinical experience in treating patients with abnormal EEG and ASD will be discussed.

Treatment of epileptiform activity on EEG in the absence of clinical seizures

There is much debate among neurologists as to the meaning of the EEG abnormalities in ASD that resemble those seen in epileptic patients. In patients who are not autistic but suffer from epilepsy, these spikes have been shown to affect cognition, sometimes language, and behavior, even when clinical seizures are not occurring (these are called interictal spikes in the absence of epileptic seizures). These interictal or subclinical spikes are similar to the spikes seen on EEG in ASD patients. There have been no formal EEG studies correlating pre- and post-treatment EEG with measured autism rating scales, language scales, or other behavioral assessment tools in a blinded or controlled manner.

I have personally collected data on treating hundreds of ASD patients with abnormal sleep EEG patterns with either various formulations of valproic acid, an anti-epileptic drug, alone or in combination with corticosteroids (either with prednisone or prednisolone orally). With treatment, I have observed a greater than 60 percent rate of EEG normalization or significant improvement in spike frequency, with correlation in receptive language performance based on clinical observation and parental reports. In 173 patients with an abnormal initial over-night abnormal EEG, 69 percent improved with just valproic acid treatment on their EEG (see Figure 20.1 for pre- and post-treatment EEG patterns). There have been case reports of reversal of autistic symptoms before, as well as smaller series of reporting improved behavior after, treatment with valproic acid in autistic children with abnormal EEG patterns without epilepsy. Other studies have reported improved behaviors with valproic acid without EEG criteria being evaluated as an outcome measure by other researchers.

Lamictal (lamotrigine), another anticonvulsant drug, has been studied in autism, but EEG abnormalities were not correlated to outcome. Interictal treat-ment of spikes in non-autistic children with lamotrigine has yielded improved behavior and cognition in a recent study from England. Another anticonvulsant, Keppra (levetiracetam), has been studied in ASD with reported improvement, but again limited data were provided about EEG and only a few cases studied in open label fashion. Single-case reports of steroid treatment or ACTH (adrenocorticotrophic hormone) therapy reversing cases of autism have been reported, but little has been noted about epilepsy or EEG in those cases.

The localization of EEG abnormalities in autistic children is different based on magnetoencephalography (MEG) reports from typically developing children with benign Rolandic-type epilepsy in at least one study. That report suggests that localization to the planum temporale or the superior surface of the left or right temporal lobe occurs, which is the same site as LKS patients' abnor-malities localize to using MEG. This is different from benign Rolandic-type of epilepsy which localizes more anteriorly along the motor cortex near the Rolandic fissure. This may be one reason why children with ASD may respond better to valproic acid, and even steroids, as these are the best medications for LKS and the epileptic phenomenon seen in that condition as well. The LKS patients also have sleep-activated epilepsy that seems to have behavioral and language aspects, as well as immune response to steroids as the treatment of choice. Despite these coincidental similarities, I agree with the majority of neu-rologists today that LKS is a different and much rarer condition than autism with regression.

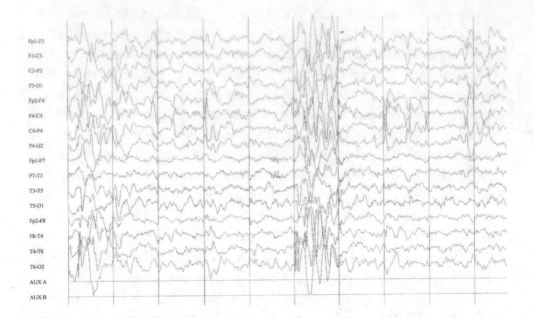

(A) Pre-treatment EEG

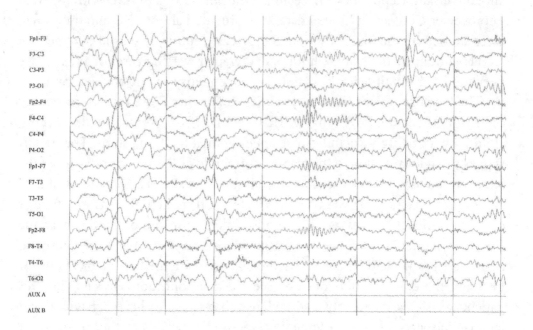

(B) Post-treatment EEG

Figure 20.1: EEG abnormality in an ASD patient before (A) and after (B) treatment with valproic acid

In autism, there can as of yet be no definitive conclusion about steroids, and of course side-effects are greater potentially than with an anticonvulsant like valproic acid. However, there is recent evidence of neuroglial inflammation in autism in brain and cerebrospinal fluid (CSF) samples, and this may be one factor that creates the epileptic spikes in this population. It may be that over many years these spikes lead to clinical epilepsy. In the 1970s and 1980s the feeling was that clinical epilepsy occurred in lower-functioning patients with ASD, and also as they got older into their teen years and early twenties clinical epilepsy became more likely. My clinical experience is that many ASD children have interictal spikes in sleep even when very young, and perhaps early treatment may prevent potential epileptic progression towards full-blown clinical seizures as these children get older. So far, the children whose EEG patterns normalized from treatment have not gone on to develop epilepsy as they have gone through later childhood and puberty. In addition to potential protection from epilepsy clinically, valproic acid may offer neuroprotection by being a mild inhibitor of interleukin 1 and interleukin 2, both found to be cytokines elevated in CSF and brain samples of autistic children studied at the Kennedy Krieger Institute at the Johns Hopkins Hospital. There is also the fact that sleep may improve and moods may stabilize with this treatment. Again, experience has shown that levels of valproic acid are best checked in the blood first thing in the morning before the morning doses are given. Behaviors are best when valproic acid levels are 90 to 120 mg/dl in the serum as the trough level.

Because of my experience with LKS, I personally do not usually choose Tegretol or Trileptol in this population as these drugs may worsen spike-wave phenomenon. However, for some teenagers and older patients with clear partial complex seizures, these drugs may be helpful. I have inherited patients on these drugs with abnormal EEG patterns who subsequently had their EEG patterns improve on valproic acid as well. Overall in the ASD population, valproic acid has been my drug of choice.

There is a rare chance of liver dysfunction, but overt liver failure is very rare, probably less than 1:50,000, or less than other drugs. Also there can be rare hematological side-effects including lowering of platelets, lower white blood cell counts, rare chances for pancreatitis, increased bruising, weight loss or weight gain, looser stools, stomach cramps, hand tremors, hair loss, and other minor side-effects. Usually valproic acid works in four to eight weeks to improve the EEG. By three to four months, a fair clinical trial should be considered as having been initiated, allowing a decision to be made about whether the medication is worth continuing based upon the clinical improvements to the patient's receptive language ability, sleep patterns, or behaviors. In addition, the EEG improvement should be evident. All of the gains should outweigh any side-effects. This is where individual clinical decisions must be made by a patient and their own physician.

Epilepsy and secondary autism

Many severe forms of early childhood epilepsy have been reported to be associated with autistic behaviors, especially if children have seizures that start before age two years. These children often have severe language dysfunction. These forms of epilepsy include Lennox-Gastaut syndrome, severe infantile myoclonus, infantile spasms, and severe cerebral palsy or hypoxic ischemic brain injury and seizures. Some studies have shown that secondary autistic characteristics have improved as seizure control is obtained through drug therapy, or even in one study treatment with the vagal nerve stimulator reducing the number of daily seizures. These children may have tens to hundreds of seizures per day and therefore differ from autism clinically where seizures are rare. Several studies in Lennox-Gastaut report improvement in behaviors, especially some autistic-type behaviors with seizure reductions. The epilepsy literature focuses mainly on seizure reduction, not autistic-like behavioral outcomes. In contrast, the literature for anticonvulsant treatment for ASD has really focused on valproic acid or lamotrigine effects on behaviors and not EEG or seizure-control outcome.

The exact mechanism of anti-epileptic drugs improving observed behaviors in these children with ASD may be directly due to improving the EEG, or perhaps by some secondary immune effect such as gamma-aminobutyric acid (GABA), anti-glutamate, N-methyl-D-aspartate (NMDA) receptor modulation, blockade of inflammatory proteins such as cytokines, or some other neuroprotective mechanism. Many anticonvulsants are also prescribed for bipolar disorders which may overlap ASD subtypes, and the clinical improvements may reflect this mode of action. It is clear that increased seizures add to poor behaviors in the secondary autism group, while the improvements seen in primary autism with anti-epileptic medications needs further study in order to clarify what mechanism is yielding the improvements.

Alternative therapies and epilepsy in ASD

Alternative practices are often quoted as saying magnesium and vitamin B6 supplementation has an anti-epileptic effect. In the many years I have been a neurologist, I have been amazed how much credence this is given by the autism alternative community. This is because pyridoxine or B6 dependent epilepsy remains very rare as a condition. I have also never seen these alternative practitioners routinely order EEG studies to evaluate for epilepsy or EEG abnormalities in their patients. In the past 16 years of my practice, I have never seen a patient taking these supplements prevented from having an abnormal EEG when they were finally screened with a 24-hour EEG. Only after appropriate treatment with medical anticonvulsants did the EEG in such patients on these supplements improve. It is my clinical observation that B6 and magnesium do not prevent this population from having abnormal EEG patterns. There have been prior reports in alternative websites quoting physiological changes; these have not documented EEG epileptic pattern changes or improved EEG, only various P300 or other evoked potential activity. Although this is interesting it does not directly address seizure potentials and treatment in the autism population.

Although no reproducible proof exists for mercury poisoning in ASD, this has not stopped parents from believing in trying chelation therapy by some alternative practitioners. In my experience, those children with abnormal EEG patterns and ASD did not have any improvement when screened after or during chelation. This again suggests no benefit from this dubious therapy. I have never seen EEG abnormalities helped by chelation therapy. Another treatment touted is vitamin methyl B12 injections. This also does not change abnormal EEG patterns in any children I have studied with 24-hour EEG who have also received that therapy.

Steroids for EEG abnormalities

Another treatment option has been with prednisone or prednisolone, often alone or in combination with valproic acid. The logic in using them was observed improvement in LKS, and the thought that there may be an improvement in EEG and language similar to the one seen in LKS. In the past 15 years, children with ASD and regression that have EEG epileptiform activity have often been referred to as LKS-variants by some neurologists studying ASD. There has been no cure in ASD from steroids in my experience using them. I also have only used them very cautiously, and perhaps in less than 2 to 3 percent of all my cases of ASD with a regression history. Subjectively noted clinical responses have been observed, however, and EEG patterns have improved in some cases where valproic acid monotherapy failed to help. This is an area of much debate, yet recent research may cause more studies to be done with steroids in the presence of abnormal EEG and possible autoimmune activity.

ACTH (adrenocorticotrophic hormone) is another steroid treatment used in epilepsy. In low doses it has helped some autistic adults and children show improved socialization. There are a few cases of autism reversal with aggressive ACTH therapy from Brazil. It has been used when rare patients cannot take oral steroids, but at this time has not been studied in any great numbers for autism cases and abnormal EEG.

Steroids are always of great potential risk, yet are often used in diseases where no other perfect treatment for autoimmune or inflammatory damage causing progression exists, such as Duchenne's muscular dystrophy, multiple sclerosis, inflammatory bowel disease, renal and pulmonary diseases, and many autoimmune diseases of children and adults. There are clear reported cases of autism where regression has occurred and been partially reversed by steroids. Series of case reports and my own experiences has shown open label experience similar to valproic acid. This has led to developing of various pulse dosing methods to minimize side-effects as well as daily protocols. These have been shown to have effects on the EEG and receptive language response in some children with ASD. In general, more research is needed, and there will be more discussion on these medications in Chapter 21 on immunology therapies in autism.

Surgical interventions for EEG abnormalities and autism

The use of subpial transaction in LKS has led some physician groups to try this surgery in rare cases of autism with regression where EEG findings show abnormalities in similar brain locations as abnormalities seen in cases of LKS. These are serious intervention treatment strategies and really ought not to be done, in my opinion in ASD cases, especially in non-convulsive cases. However, there are some case reports of EEG improvement after the technique. This again raises the question of whether the EEG spikes are being treated or the actual disorder. At this time no one actively believes there is a surgical option for these types of cases. I do not know of any reversal of the underlying autism by this method of intervention.

Conclusion

The current state of the art in neurology does not have an agreed treatment protocol for abnormal EEG patterns in ASD in the absence of clinical seizures.

Future research should focus on neuroprotective aspects of this early treatment. Perhaps early treatment before clinical epilepsy becomes manifest would prevent the current trend for increased risk of epilepsy as children with ASD get older. Again, this is something that has to be studied. The best way for progress to be made is to obtain early EEG screening in this population, and then randomize and study both treatment and natural course in the ASD subpopulation with abnormal EEG patterns. More research is currently being done on the immune aspects of glial inflammation and autism; this may yield better understanding linking immunology and epileptic patterns that may be part of the disease process making up what we are seeing in ASD. This may help to explain the abnormal EEG patterns, which will ultimately lead to better treatments. More research is needed, but at this time, valproic acid is my favorite medication for treating the types of EEG abnormalities observed in ASD. Steroids are only to be used in rare cases with clear regression patterns and immune history perhaps. Alternative therapies at this time clearly do not address EEG and epilepsy in autism.

Chapter 21

Immunological Medical Therapy

Prior chapters have discussed the theories of immunology and neuroglial inflammation in autism and autistic spectrum disorders (ASD). This is currently a very exciting area where new research and potential therapies are advancing and may offer new hopes of prevention and treatment. This could provide the common environmental link between genetics and environmental triggers in ASD, and may explain the trend of increasing numbers of cases over the past 15 years. This chapter will review the treatment options currently available and some perhaps on the horizon.

Immunoglobulin therapy

Immunoglobulin therapy is based on the theory that some autistic children have mild forms of immunodeficiency. This has been clinically based on observations of their getting recurrent illnesses of otitis media or upper respiratory type infections, and perhaps having lower levels of total serum IgG, IgA, or IgG subtypes of immunoglobulin proteins in their blood when tested. Perhaps 25 to 30 percent of autistic children may have mild deficiencies, and perhaps 60 percent get recurrent infections as mentioned above. There are also increased rates of chronic diarrhea. This has led some physicians to treat with intravenous infusions of immunoglobulins or IVIG.

IVIG is protein from human blood product that is pharmacologically produced and has been purified against being contaminated with infections such as the AIDS virus (HIV) and hepatitis. This is given in doses of 400 mg/kg to 1000 mg/kg per dose every month for three to six doses. The patient is then observed to see if autistic symptoms improve. This theoretically would shut down and suppress internal autoimmune antibody production and change T-cell ratios of helper to suppressor ratios. There is a reported 10 percent rate of improvement in two open label non-placebo controlled studies in autism. This treatment is very costly, perhaps $5000–$10,000 per treatment, and some insurers do not pay unless purely for immune deficiency that must be clinically documented. There have been rare allergic reactions to this since it is a protein infusion. Also, this can in rare cases cause stress from fluid load on the kidneys and heart. This therapy is seldom done, but has been popular at times in the past due to television talkshow exposures and occasional case reports. This has not been that useful in epilepsy where it has been studied, nor in PANDAS diseases where some obsessive-compulsive disorder (OCD) symptoms are autoimmune in nature. There is not good evidence showing how this affects the central nervous system glial inflammation system.

Steroids

Steroids that have been used in ASD comprise mainly the oral agents prednisone and prednisolone. They have been used in autism based on a few case reports, and one case sensationalized on television in the early 1990s. That case was a boy with autistic regression but a normal electroencephalogram (EEG) who showed steroid response to regain his receptive language and then some expressive language.

There have been many cases of autism with abnormal EEG patterns, but none meeting clinical criteria for Landau-Kleffner syndrome (LKS), that have had partial responses to steroid therapy. Some clinical case reports and series of pulse dose cases have been published. Unfortunately, there have been no placebo-controlled medical studies to date, but open label experience shows increased language receptively and expressively more verbal output with increased single and multiple word usages overall.

In my own experience, perhaps 2 to 3 percent of patients in my practice with clinical histories of regression and autism who also have abnormal EEG patterns in sleep have been given either daily or pulse dosing protocols for prednisone or prednisolone. Many children in my practice first got three to six months of anticonvulsant therapy, and then if all parties felt only a partial clinical or EEG recovery was made, the parents and I would discuss adding on a trial of prednisone or oral prednisolone as either daily or pulse therapy. I predominantly used pulse dosing of prednisone, and this resulted in fewer Cushenoid side-effects. Cushenoid effects are the steroidal weight gain with central fat deposits, puffy face, bloating, and potentials for increased blood pressure and weight gain. Also elevated blood sugars, cataracts, skin stretch marks, stomach stress ulcers, and lower resistance to infection can occur with steroid therapy. Since there can be risk for infection, opportunistic community infections can occur and potentially serious side-effects and even serious infections can be seen in any case where the immune system is suppressed. Great caution must be exercised by anyone using these medications. Each physician should have their own policy and methods for safely managing steroids in their patients. Many physicians may never feel comfortable with these medications. I cannot say that steroids must be tried in every child with autism. However, in some select cases they may be worth a try if the quality-of-life issues are severely affected by a loss of skills and there is enough EEG evidence for a case similar to a LKS type regression, or strong case for a post-infectious or autoimmune history with clinical regression pre-dating the onset of an ASD. Every patient and physician must evaluate each case individually. Recommended steroid doses that have been reported as useful for prednisone have ranged from 1 to 3 mg/kg per day as the initial daily dose or pulse dosing twice weekly with 5 to 10 mg/kg. Again each case may require individual modification.

There have also been cases of inflammatory bowel disease and nephritic kidney disease in autistic individuals where high-dose prednisone therapy reversed concurrent autism. In no way should these dosages be used as anything but a range of what has been used in the literature or prior case reports. This book is not recommending any specific therapeutic method and is not to be used as a medical textbook to guide therapy. This is merely summarizing prior experiences. Until controlled series of research studies are available, this is the best information to date on this issue.

Other immune therapies

The inhibition of B and T cells can be accomplished by other drugs. For some immune vasculitis cases, the chemotherapeutic agent methotrexate has been used, as well as 6-mercaptopurine for inflammatory bowel disease. These are sometimes used in cases of Crohn's disease and in concurrent cases of autism there have been reported improvements in some of these children. There has been a small open label trial of thalidomide at 50 mg per day with clinical global improvement in 3/6 children with treatment for four months but this was not continued longer for fear of side-effects.

Thalidomide may inhibit tumor necrosis factor-alpha and other autoimmune factors in chronic inflammation. Other drugs that may inhibit tumor necrosis factor-alpha include Enbrel (etanercept) and Remicade (infliximab), both injections; but to date none have been formally studied in ASD. Turmeric is currently being studied as a nutritional supplement that may have anti-inflammatory properties that may inhibit tumor necrosis factor-alpha. Another herbal remedy that inhibits tumor necrosis factor-alpha is the herb cat's claw (*uña de gato*) from South America. Unfortunately these are just being studied in open label pilot trials and have not yet been published to date in ASD.

There is effort to use low-dose Trexan (naltrexone) on the theory this drug may alter the effect of endorphins on activating inflammation and may cause modified ratios of T-helper to T-suppressor type cells. So far this has only open label anecdotal data, but warrants further research.

Researchers are currently developing drugs that inhibit neurogial in the central nervous system but leave peripheral immune function alone. Plasmapharesis has been used in PANDAS cases of post-streptococcal OCD but has not been used widely in ASD. Agents that may affect cytokine inflammation may be useful in the future. It may be necessary to begin doing lumbar puncture studies of cerebrospinal fluid (CSF) in order to screen and design future therapies of immunomodulation for ASD in the future.

Currently no single immune therapy is clinically recommended for ASD. If strongly suspected, discuss immune history issues with your physician, consider doing spinal fluid studies and even looking for research centers studying neuroglial inflammation in autism, which as of today represent no more than three centers in the United States. Despite this lack of definitive therapy currently, the future may very well lie here for prevention and reversal of many autism issues.

Chapter 22

Gastrointestinal Issues

Autistic spectrum patients have systemic problems that often get confusing labels from alternative practitioners, such as "sensory integration disorder" and "leaky gut disorder." These non-specific terms often mislead parents who are confused by histories of diarrhea or constipation in their children and who feel they are not supported by their family doctor or pediatricians. The problem is that neurologically impaired children, especially those prone to stress and anxiety, poor attention, and poor sensory input to pain, may become encoporetic (severely constipated or impacted by stool withholding), and sometimes also have irritable bowel, which is often a comorbid condition in psychiatric conditions like obsessive-compulsive disorder (OCD) and anxiety disorders. Children with attention deficit disorder or cerebral palsy also have these complications. However, in autism a whole economy has sprung up with laboratory testing of stool samples, names like pancreatic insufficiency, leaky gut, dysbiosis (abnormal gut flora), yeast infection, gluten-casein sensitivity, and other terms that have convinced parents that their children have serious gastrointestinal problems causing brain problems. The term "gut–brain syndrome" has been coined.

The truth is that most of these diagnoses are made without any official pediatric gastroenterology specialists examining or doing appropriate testing in these children. In fact, there has been a lack of interest in appropriate medical evaluation of these children's gastrointestinal complaints in the past, so that just recently gastroenterologists are beginning to address some of these issues scientifically in the autistic spectrum disorder (ASD) population. My clinical view is that the gastrointestinal issues in ASD are secondary to, and not the primary cause of, the brain issues. This chapter will discuss the known facts that have been found regarding the comorbid gut issues in ASD.

Gastrointestinal symptoms

Autistic patients often present with histories of being picky eaters and frequently crave carbohydrates and such food. The parents sometimes believe they are "addicted" to gluten and casein from the hype that is out in the lay literature. This is not true. Often these are imprinted toddler foods that are easy to chew with the associated poor oral motor strength and dyspraxia these children have. Also these children have chronic loose stools or alternating diarrhea or constipation. Many times there is a family history of this, as well as sometimes of irritable bowel. Certainly family history is important, especially if there is one of celiac sprue or Crohn's inflammatory bowel disease. There is also another disease more recently being diagnosed called eosinophilic gastroenteritis presenting with failure to thrive and infantile onset of food allergies and intolerances that may overlap pervasive developmental disorders (PDD) as well. These issues should prompt appropriate referral to a gastrointestinal pediatric specialist. Common problems do present more often in ASD patients than others, and these should be considered by pediatricians.

Strange irritability, screaming, or posturing may represent gastroesophageal reflux disease. There may be chewing or bad breath with this as well. Sometimes I have even seen ASD children pull their teeth or eat strange things to counteract this type of pain. Also some researchers have found increased evidence of lactose intolerance in autistic individuals compared to controls. Bloating and extra flatus or loose stools after dairy may be a clue, as well as family history. The other common oversight is not looking for constipation as the cause of diarrhea, called overflow diarrhea. I call this the "rocks in the river" problem. Basically the children get blocked with hard stool and only looser stool can get around. The evaluation should include a basic physical exam of the abdomen, a rectal exam by your doctor, and an x-ray of the abdomen called an abdominal flat plate or KUB (kidney-ureter-bladder) film. This test often shows excessive stool content and can be treated by laxatives and a cleanout procedure for the bowel. In my experience this is a common cause of so-called diarrhea in this population.

These basic pediatric care issues should be done before expensive alternative testing or stool cultures are done. Therefore every child should have a basic evaluation for their intestinal complaints by their pediatric doctor to look for reflux, constipation, and possible food intolerances, including thinking of lactose intolerance, if the symptoms fit. Multiple medications for gastroesophageal reflux are available and can be prescribed by pediatricians and gastroenterologists for this common condition. For constipation, many laxatives, including senna, Miralax, mineral oil, aloe vera, and other remedies, are available. Always work with your physician for the best treatment plan to help your child's chronic constipation issues.

Gluten/casein-free diet

In my experience the gluten/casein-free diet has not made a major impact in ASD patients. This diet does not specifically address celiac disease, and the majority of patients I have seen have not had any evidence of milk or gluten sensitivity. In the rare true celiac sprue cases I have seen with autism, the gastrointestinal symptoms did get better on the diet, but the autism did not really improve. There are laboratory tests for anti-gliadin antibodies for IgG and IgA. There is also a test for tissue transglutamase (TTG) which is specific for celiac sprue. Intestinal biopsy is the ultimate diagnostic test. This has rarely been done in patients I have seen with ASD on this type of diet. When a biopsy has been obtained, it is usually normal.

In most ASD patients I have examined who had tried the gluten/casein-free diet, they may have had elevated anti-gliadin IgG levels, but not TTG or IgA anti-gliadin levels. It is my opinion that the IgG levels are not specific and cross-react with other autoimmune issues. Other wheat and milk allergy testing has usually been normal. I have not personally seen what is reported as helpful in the alternative literature. Ongoing research has yet to show definitive help in core autistic features from this diet. What parents may be seeing is a placebo effect, or perhaps because of a lower total or perhaps more complex type of carbohydrate diet the children may not be getting as hyperactive as on a more typical simple high-carbohydrate diet. Similar changes have been reported with Feingold diets for hyperactivity, and the ketogenic diet for epilepsy. I do not recommend this diet to my patients and in fact recommend a lower total carbohydrate diet instead. If celiac sprue is suspected then an appropriate work-up is in order.

Secretin

The story of this drug is probably one of the most interesting chapters in autism history. There are still believers despite multiple trials and double-blind placebo-controlled trials showing lack of effect. This started after television hysteria about this pancreatic-stimulating drug that when given intravenously to stimulate pancreatic secretions for endoscopic testing caused lasting speech effects in autistic children. Little credence was given to the possible effect of the anesthetic given prior to the procedure, or the fact that a colonic cleanout was given before the test, which may have alleviated chronic discomfort. This led to massive claims and hysteria to give secretin to autistic children.

This drug caused some patients to have hyperactive and tic behaviors, and caused worsened diarrhea in others. In multiple controlled studies no definite benefits were found, and yet alternative practitioners are still offering this as treatment, even as topical transdermal creams (which when analyzed in one case had no secretin content).

Again, this whole aspect was another example of the desperation of a treatment being promoted by alternative treatment groups before scientific facts could support the validity. This is similar to the chelation issues now in the media. *Caveat emptor* remains the important legacy of secretin. I do not think anyone should be prescribing this drug.

Chapter 23

Medications for Core Symptoms of Language and Behavior

Autism impairs most dramatically at the levels of social and communication abilities. There is currently no official treatment to cure this disorder. There is growing evidence that speech and frontal lobe processing regions are impaired in the autistic brain vs. controls. There is evidence that epileptiform and inflammatory activity may damage some of these regions of brain function. This chapter will focus on my clinical experience using medications to improve different aspects of communication as a way to improve the core deficits in autistic patients and therefore improve their quality of functional life.

Receptive language: Presence of abnormal EEG

This is not an area all neurologists agree on, as previously mentioned in this book. However, I feel that if the patient has abnormal spike or spike-wave activity present in sleep over the temporal-parietal or temporal central regions even in the absence of clinical epilepsy, they warrant a trial of Depakote (valproic acid). This drug has shown approximately a 70 percent improvement rate in electroencephalogram (EEG) pattern normalization as well as improvement in receptive speech processing. This is in my opinion a good first step when the patient has an abnormal EEG. Before other medications are tried, it helps to control this aspect of the brain disorder. This is especially true when other behavior medications are needed that may lower seizure resistance thresholds, such as the antipsychotic medications, or perhaps antidepressants. Once a trial of treating the abnormal EEG is complete and the degree of language recovery is assessed, the following medications can still be tried in addition. The usual trial period for assessing the valproic acid treatment in my experience is eight to twelve weeks with the goal of keeping trough level at 90 to 120 mg/dl.

Receptive and expressive language: Medications after EEG treatment or normal EEG

The next phase of receptive speech help that has been studied includes three classes of therapy: L-carnosine, a dipeptide nutritional supplement; donezepil (Aricept), Razadyne (galantamine), and rivastigmine (Exelon), cholinesterase inhibitors and Alzheimer's medications; and memantine (Namenda, Ebixa), an N-methyl-D-aspartate (NMDA)/glutamate blocker and Alzheimer medication. These have all been studied with either open label or placebo-controlled studies in autism and have shown improvements in core symptoms of language and behavior.

L-carnosine is a natural dipeptide that is found in the brain and also acts as a neuroprotective protein in the enterorhinal frontal cortex and mesiotemporal brain regions where it can block excess copper and zinc influx during cellular inflammation and ischemia. L-carnosine may also act as an anti-oxidant protective supplement in the brain. A double-blind placebo-controlled study has been published showing improved behavior and receptive language processing in autism. Irritability can occur in 20 to 30 percent of cases, but no other physical side-effects have been seen. A rare metabolic disorder, carnosinase deficiency, can cause hypercarnosinemia, which can occur in 1:4000 births. This can be a contraindication to using carnosine.

Aricept (donezepil) is a long-acting acetyl cholinesterase inhibitor that increases acetyl choline in the frontal lobes. This may be deficient in the parietal and frontal cortical connections in autism, according to work in autism, and has been shown in open label and placebo-controlled studies to improve behavior and receptive language with some expressive language improvement in 50–60 percent of treated autistic children. Exelon (rivastigmine) is a shorter-duration mixed cholinesterase inhibitor that in an open label study showed effect upon receptive and expressive language and improved behavior and slightly improved attention. Side-effects have included irritability in 30 percent and gastrointestinal problems in 10 to 20 percent.

Memantine (Namenda, Ebixa are trade names) is a drug that is an antagonist to NMDA receptors and glutamate receptors that may play a role in both epilepsy, brain neurogenesis, learning, and end stage neuroglial inflammation.

All of these pathways may be important in autism. Over 400 children with autism have been treated with this drug and over 70 percent have shown improved social behavior and interests, and better receptive and expressive language efforts; many have seen better motor processing with dyspraxia. Only 10 to 15 percent have shown irritability or manic behavior exacerbation and no other physical side-effects have been noted, even with concurrent polytherapy. More studies are currently underway. Cycloserine, in a small series of ten patients, also acting as a weaker NMDA antagonist, has also shown some global improvement in autism in an open label study from Indiana University. There is basic scientific evidence that glutamate and NMDA receptors may be important in autistic brain regulation. Another NMDA antagonist called amantidine has also shown some positive effects in a single placebo-controlled study.

Steroids and other hormones

Corticosteroids like prednisone have been reported periodically to help speech and language recovery in autistic individuals. This has been discussed in chapters on immune therapy; however, there are reports of ACTH (adrenocorticotrophic hormone) injections at levels of two or three units per day equivalents being used in adults and children in England having some effect on social awareness and empathy. In addition, oxytocin has been given as a hormone that is similar to pitocin at labor and delivery. This hormone has shown increased social empathy in autistic adults in open label use. Prednisone use has been shown to increase language and change abnormal EEG patterns and reverse regressive cases in this population based on open label case reports. The side-effects of steroids always need to be carefully monitored and should, in my opinion, only be given in rare cases.

Conclusion

Despite a lack of conclusive research, there are many medications that can be used to improve core receptive language and also affect to some degree expressive and social language behaviors. Currently, my best experience has been with memantine, the supplement L-carnosine, and valproic acid for those patients with abnormal EEG patterns of central-temporal or generalized types. Further research may lead to more conclusive uses for these medication options. In addition, anti-inflammatory medications may alter autistic spectrum disorder (ASD) symptoms in the future. Again, always consult your physician to discuss any treatment options in ASD.

Chapter 24

A Rational Approach to Medical Treatment
Case Studies

The purpose of this chapter is to give examples of how to work up and put to use the knowledge contained in this book. Through theoretical cases based on clinical prototypes seen over the years in my pediatric neurology practice, I will illustrate how to work up and decide on treatment choices in a given patient. There is no one correct answer, and these examples are merely to show you the thought process I use in my clinic. Your physician may guide you differently and can certainly use these examples to explain why his point of view may be different from this author. That is the point of this book, providing a meeting ground to discuss a rational approach to intervene actively to make medical decisions to improve the quality of life for autistic patients.

Case 1: Autism/No regression/No sleep

History: This was a four-year-old male with chronic history of problems getting to sleep, hyperactivity all day long, and waking two or three times for hours at night. He was constantly on the go and had limited single echolalia words for expressive speech and seemed to understand simple single commands but not two- or three-step commands. He was not yet toilet trained, and he had a history of loose stools. He was a full-term pregnancy with unremarkable delivery first born child. He was an irritable baby from day one and was always hyperactive. He never made good eye contact, never pointed or had language. He never regressed.

A prior neurologist had tried Ritalin at age three and he became aggressive and seemed to hallucinate and scream all day, then not sleep for 36 hours. He has been on the gluten/casein-free diet with no help.

Decision point: Categorize autism type: non-regressive/no language/manic/poor sleep/gastrointestinal issues.

Plan: After the initial consultation I obtained an electroencephalogram (EEG) to evaluate sleep and manic issues as well as language reception. This was normal. A magnetic resonance image (MRI) was not obtained. He was started on tizanidine for sleep initiation and valproic acid for manic behaviors. A kidney-ureter-bladder (KUB) film was ordered to rule out chronic constipation. He had diffuse increased stool and dilated loops of colon and was started on Miralax daily which helped normalize and increase the size and output of his stool. He had better sleep onset with tizanidine, and once valproic acid levels were titrated to steady state of 110 mg/dl his behavior became calmer and his sleep improved. He still has occasional breakthrough periods of agitation. Considerations include possible trials of additional Risperdal or similar medication next. He has been tapered from the gluten/casein-free diet with no change or worsening in behaviors. He will not go back to drinking milk on his own.

Discussion: This case shows how stimulants may exacerbate mania and hyperactivity may respond poorly in autism. The gluten/casein-free diet had no positive effect and actually caused him not to like dairy foods, therefore limiting his current protein intake. Treating his sleep and gastrointestinal issues appropriately helped quality of life, although he still has limited communication and is lower functioning. His EEG was normal, and valproic acid was chosen for bipolar behavioral issues not EEG treatment. An atypical antipsychotic medication may still need to be added.

Case 2: Autistic female with seizures

History: This was an eight-year-old with uncomplicated pregnancy induced by fertility drugs that after full-term delivery had a normal neonatal period. She had a quiet infancy with slow normal motor development, walking by 17 months, but speech was delayed until after three years and she always had poor eye contact. She had a large head and atypical poor fine motor skills. Her normal to large head size was felt familial. No prior genetic work-up was done. Seizures began age three years with partial complex staring spells and turning head to the left with stiffening and staring. EEG showed mild abnormal slowing only. Failed multiple medications and seizures have worsened. Behavioral outbursts of aggression have occurred periodically. Unusual periodic episodes of hyperventilation have been occurring for past three years, attributed to anxiety but when witnessed during visit no obvious behavioral aspect noted. MRI of her brain was normal in the past, and she was seen by several neurologists.

Decision point: Hyperventilation, worsening seizures. This child has worsening seizures despite several medications, and perhaps a diagnosis has been missed with her breathing episodes perhaps being part of Rett's syndrome, even though she lacks the classic full developmental arrest and the midline hand self-stimulations.

Plan: She was given a chromosome test for Rett's syndrome that came back positive. Her seizure medications were maximized. Parents were referred appropriately to specialists in Rett's syndrome and for genetic counseling.

Case 3: Regression age 15 months/Male with sleep disturbances

History: A normal-appearing three-year-old child with normal birth was born in good health after a full-term pregnancy. Infancy was normal to advanced with walking by ten months of age and words for "mama, dada, dog, his sister, and milk" by 13 months of age. He also pointed and waved. This child started having multiple ear infections and was on several courses of antibiotics by 18 months of age, receiving ear tubes by his second birthday. No documented hearing loss was measured, but by 18 months he seemed not to respond to calling his name or language, yet knew television or other sounds. He seemed to be less responsive after 15 months. He was noted to stare off for brief periods of time, and sleep changed from sleeping through the night to waking around 1am to 2am several nights per week, crying and having trouble going back to sleep. He became more withdrawn, stopped pointing, started to line up toys and flap his hands by age two years. No other problems were known.

Decision point: History regression, loss of language skills, sleep disturbances and staring episodes, acts deaf.

Plan: This child is one who needs a work-up for an overnight EEG. He also needs careful neurological examination to rule out any sign of a degenerative motor or focal physical finding. Possible degenerative diseases need to be in the differential, but most likely this is a regressive autism subtype. The overnight EEG came back abnormal with fairly common but not continuous spike-wave discharges over the right temporal-parietal region with some generalized spread during sleep. Awake activity, including noted staring or self-stimulatory episodes, were non-epileptic in the EEG tracing. Valproic acid was started and the child after three weeks finally got to a high therapeutic range and sleep improved. After nine weeks his language reception got better. He began sleeping through the night after only three weeks of valproic acid. He returned to the clinic after 12 weeks and had a repeat overnight EEG that showed rare transient right temporal lobe slow rhythmic asymmetric activity in sleep only. No definite epileptiform activity was seen. Receptive speech was better, and he was naming many more items with flash cards in his applied behavioral analysis (ABA) therapy sessions. Memantine was added and he was seen eight weeks later and had increased receptive speech, had progressed even more in ABA therapy, his expressive speech was showing one- to three-word spontaneous utterances, and he was socially interested in being around other children in the same room for the first time. Sleep continued to be stable. An MRI of the brain was obtained and was normal.

Discussion: This child showed EEG improvement and also there was no structural damage evident on the MRI of the brain as is typical in these cases. The speech and sleep improved and some degree of language and social core symptoms improved with therapy. This child represents the prototype of ASD with regression and abnormal sleep EEG that has primary language regression. Core language and social symptoms can improve to some degree with this regimen. Each individual needs their own assessment and individualized medication plan.

Case 4: Patient with Asperger's

History: A 12-year-old male with intellectually superior functioning with verbal intelligence quotient (IQ) score of 139, but performance score of 112.

He has very good standardized scores especially in math, but some trouble with spelling. No history of seizure activity in the past. Language was slow until age three, when it came on fluently. Toilet training was normal. He always obsessed about dinosaurs, cartoon trading cards, trains, and United States presidents. Currently he is very interested only in college basketball team statistics. He is very good with computers. He has no real friends. He sleeps fine, has no gastro-intestinal issues. He is very distractible. Last semester he did no homework because he saw no point to it as it was "boring," got low grades in his classes, because he was playing a computer game online in his spare time. He denies being depressed or anxious. There are no obvious obsessive-compulsive disorder (OCD) issues.

Decision point: This patient has no seizure or language fluency issues. I typically do not get an EEG in Asperger's patients. This patient has inconsistent performance and distractibility. He has no current anxiety or excessive compulsive or obsessive traits. There are no psychotic or manic traits. His school issues require help focusing his attention.

Discussion: This patient would most likely benefit from a trial of a stimulant or non-stimulant approach to attention deficit disorder (ADD). These patients are not usually the hyperactive subtypes of ADD. Unlike autism, Asperger's patients do respond well to medications for ADD in general. If overly obsessed on a topic, a selective serotonin reuptake inhibitor (SSRI) may also be added later

Case 5: Late autistic regression/Abnormal EEG/
Autoimmune family history

History: A three-year-old male with history of normal speech in one- and two-word sentences by age 15 to 18 months. He was living in France and spoke both English and French. Waving and gesturing and pointing were present. The child had a high fever of 104 Fahrenheit with a viral illness and had what was felt to be a febrile seizure of generalized nature at 19 months of age. He was obtunded (not responsive, lethargic) immediately afterwards and did not really talk after this illness for several weeks. At the time no evidence was felt by the family or pediatrician that the child had meningitis or encephalitis. No lumbar puncture was done. The child lost all speech, started to run around and no longer responded to calling out his name. The child had occasional blank staring spells and acted as if he were deaf. He lost eye contact. Sometimes he would flap his hands when excited or stressed. Sleep became disrupted. No EEG was performed. The child was given speech and ABA therapy and minimal responsiveness was noted. Family history is significant for autoimmune thyroiditis in a maternal aunt and severe psoriasis and rheumatoid arthritis in the paternal family.

Decision point: This patient had a very late sudden regression following a viral illness. He needs a metabolic work-up to rule out a genetic or metabolic disorder that could be triggered by stress of a fever. He also needs an autoimmune work-up for possible autoimmune disease. He needs an epilepsy work-up and neuroimaging evaluation as well. Lumbar puncture was also performed on this child.

The metabolic testing was negative for mitochondrial and organic or amino acidurias. The lumbar puncture was negative for metabolic abnormalities, but did show neuroglial activation (research laboratory collaboration) and elevated tumor necrosis factor. Peripheral blood showed low immunoglobulins and low IgA levels, and presence of an anti-endothelial capillary antibody. The EEG showed very active bilateral independent sleep-activated temporal-central polyspike-wave discharges in sleep. His MRI of the brain was normal.

Discussion: The patient responded to dramatic receptive speech and return of expressive single words with valproic acid. Later prednisone and carnosine were added and further language and behavioral changes were noted. Memantine was later added with only slight improvement. After the low IgA and IgG levels were found, four courses of intravenous immunoglobulin were given and the prednisone pulse dosing tapered down. This caused another jump in his recovery. His EEG is now normalized after one year of therapy, and he has good receptive speech, but very delayed expressive speech still. He is still in the autistic diagnosis category, but his eye contact, receptive responsiveness, and toy and social skill interests have moved closer to normal.

Case 6: Female with ischemic encephalopathy/ Seizures/Autistic variant

History: This is a five-year-old patient that had a prolonged labor and vacuum-assisted delivery after an uneventful full-term pregnancy. The child probably had seizures that went unnoticed as a newborn, and after going home was having stiffening spells and screaming episodes throughout infancy.

Despite the mother's efforts, the child's pediatricians did not feel anything was wrong. Language started but was atypical. The child never slept more than one or two hours at a time. She had frequent staring spells. She had unusual words, but none for "mama." Everyone thought she was a genius because of intricate block designs she would make. She was very hyperactive. She was aggressive. She went to a famous teaching hospital and was labeled one of the worst 10 percent of autistic children they had seen, predicting future institutionalization. A trial of Prozac made her very manic. Family history shows bipolar disease and autoimmune disease and autism in the paternal family and anxiety and OCD in the maternal family. The child would go 48 hours with no more than one or two hours of sleep.

Decision point: This child required an overnight EEG that showed bitemporal spike-wave with secondary generalized polyspike discharges during sleep. She was started on Depakote with improved speech and behavior, but was still very manic and not sleeping. Risperdal caused a dystonic reaction and she was placed on Seroquel and also tizanidine for sleep. She eventually slept through the night. Later she was started on Memantine and had improved speech and motor planning and stopped toe walking. She also continued to have OCD and panic symptoms and at times became depressed. A low dose of Effexor was added and this helped her moods. She had terrible attention span but could tolerate any medication for attention without becoming more manic.

Discussion: This case illustrates complex interaction of polypharmacy in a very manic patient with underlying seizures from an early age with resulting autistic behaviors and OCD and anxiety as well. Treating her underlying seizures and manic condition allowed great improvement in her quality of life and allowed her not to be institutionalized. She is more a mixture of secondary autism with multiple predisposing risk factors environmentally and genetically.

Conclusions

The case studies shown in this chapter are examples of how these patients are part of a broad spectrum and need individualized care. Each patient needs the full neurological evaluation and clinical knowledge applied to their individual situation. I often explain to my patients this is part detective work sorting out the facts of an individual case, part like building a house—needing to start at the foundation of the problems first, then layering on the treatment—and part like repairing a sophisticated computer with tape (imagine a computer chip repair).

Our current knowledge is limited, and there are no cures; but more and more, biological interventions can improve the quality of life for these patients. Researchers are giving us more clues into what genetically and environmentally may be causing this epidemic. We have to clinically treat the deficits these children have now. The current drugs and how to use them are only templates for the reader to use as a guide in conjunction with their own physician. If the reader is a medical professional, use this book to stimulate how to improve on your approach in intervening effectively for these patients. Goals should be to improve the core symptoms of communication and social function, but not neglect basic care like sleep or epilepsy or gastrointestinal care. I hope this book will be a catalyst for that type of help.

One day I hope I can write a definitive book for the cure or prevention of this devastating disorder.

Bibliography

Chapter I

American Academy of Pediatrics (2001) 'The pediatrician's role in the diagnosis and management of autistic spectrum disorder in children.' *Pediatrics 107*, 1221–1226.

Baron-Cohen, S., Allen, J., and Gillberg, C. (1992) 'Can autism be detected at 18 months? The needle, the haystack, and the CHAT.' *British Journal of Psychiatry 161*, 839–843.

Garnett, M.S. and Attwood, A.J. (1998) 'The Australian Scale for Asperger's Syndrome.' In T. Attwood (ed) *Asperger's Syndrome: A Guide for Parents and Professionals* (pp.17–19). London: Jessica Kingsley Publishers.

Goldman, S., Salgado, M., Wang, C., Kim, M., Greene, P., and Rapin, I. (2005) 'Motor stereotypies in autistic versus non-autistic preschool developmental disabilities.' *Annals of Neurology 58*, Suppl 9, S88–90 (Abstract).

Kanner, L. (1943) 'Autistic disturbances of affective contact.' *Nervous Child 10*, 217–250.

Miller, J.M., Singer, H.S., Bridges, D.D., and Waranch, H.R. (2006) 'Behavioral therapy for treatment of stereotypic movements in non-autistic children.' *Journal of Child Neurology 21*, 2, 119–125.

Myles, B., Bock, S., and Simpson, R. (2000) *Asperger Symptom Diagnostic Scale.* Austin, TX: Pro-Ed Inc.

Schieve, L.A., Rice, C., Boyle, C., Visser, S.N., and Blumberg, S.J. (2006) 'Mental health in the United States: Parental report of diagnosed autism in children aged 4–17 years—United States, 2003–2004. *Morbidity and Mortality Weekly Report 55*, 17, 481–486.

Siegel, B. (1998) 'Early screening and diagnosis in autistic spectrum disorders: The Pervasive Developmental Disorders Screening Test (PDDST).' Presented at the National Institute of Health State of Science on Autism Screening and Working Conference, Bethesda, MD, June 15–17.

Stone, W.L., Coonrod, E.E., and Ousley, O.Y. (2000) 'Brief report: Screening Tool for Autism in Two-year-olds (STAT), Development and preliminary data.' *Journal of Autism Developmental Disorders 30*, 607–612.

Chapter 2

Filipek, P.A., Accardo, P.J., Ashwal, S., *et al.* (2000) 'Practice parameter: Screening and diagnosis of autism.' Report of the Quality Standards Subcommittee of the American Academy of Neurology and Child Neurology Society. *Neurology 55*, 469–479.

Lord, C., Risi, S., DiLavore, P.S., Shulman, C., Thurm, A., and Pickles, A. (2006) 'Autism from 2 to 9 years.' *Archives of General Psychiatry 63*, 694–701.

Chapter 3

American Psychiatric Association (2000) *Diagnostic and Statistical Manual of Mental Disorders* (4th edition, text revised). Washington, DC: American Psychiatric Association.

Baird, G., Charman, T., Baron-Cohen, S., *et al.* (2000) 'A screening instrument for autism at 18 months of age: A 6-year follow-up study.' *Journal of the American Academy of Child and Adolescent Psychiatry 40*, 1457–1463.

Garnett, M.S. and Attwood, A.J. (1998) 'The Australian Scale for Asperger's Syndrome.' In T. Attwood (ed) *Asperger's Syndrome: A Guide for Parents and Professionals* (pp.17–19). London: Jessica Kingsley Publishers.

Gilliam, J.E. (1995) *Gilliam Autism Rating Scale (GARS)*. Austin, TX: Pro-Ed Inc.

Lord, C., Risi, S., DiLavore, P.S., Shulman, C., Thurm, A., and Pickles, A. (2006) 'Autism from 2 to 9 years.' *Archives of General Psychiatry 63*, 694–701.

Lord, C., Risi, S., Lambrecht, L., *et al.* (2000) 'The Autism Diagnostic Schedule—Generic: A standard measure of social and communication deficits associated with the spectrum of autism.' *Journal of Autism Developmental Disorders 30*, 205–223.

Lord, C., Rutter, M., and LeConteur, A. (1994) 'Autism Diagnostic Interview—Revised: A revised version of a diagnostic interview for caregivers of individuals with possible pervasive developmental disorders.' *Journal of Autism Developmental Disorders 24*, 659–685.

Myles, B., Bock, S., and Simpson, R. (2000) *Asperger Syndrome Diagnostic Scale*. Austin, TX: Pro-Ed Inc.

Schopler, E., Reichler, R.J., DeVellis, R.F., *et al.* (1980) 'Toward objective classification of childhood autism: Childhood Autism Ratings Scale (CARS).' *Journal of Autism Developmental Disorders 10*, 91–103.

Chapter 4

Chez, M.G., Buchanan, C., Loeffel, M., *et al.* (1998) 'Treatment of electroencephalographic epileptiform activity on overnight EEG studies in children with pervasive developmental disorder or autism: defining similarities to the Landau-Kleffner syndrome.' *Journal of Developmental Learning Disorders 2*, 217–229.

Gillberg, C. and Coleman, M. (1992) *The Biology of the Autistic Syndromes.* London: Mac Keith Press.

Gilberg, C. and Coleman, M. (1994) 'Autism and medical disorders: A review of the literature.' *Developmental Medicine and Child Neurology 36*, 50–56.

Piven, J., Gayle, J., Landa, R., *et al.* (1991) 'The prevalence of Fragile X in a sample of autistic individuals diagnosed using a standardized interview.' *Journal of the American Academy of Child Adolescent Psychiatry 30*, 825–830.

Spence, S.J. (2004) 'The genetics of autism.' *Seminars in Pediatric Neurology 11*, 196–204.

Tuchman, R.F. and Rapin, I. (1997) 'Regression in pervasive developmental disorders: Seizures and epileptiform electroencephalogram correlates.' *Pediatrics 99*, 560–566.

Wassink, T.H., Piven, J., and Patil, S.R. (2001) 'Chromosomal abnormalities in a clinic sample of individuals with autistic disorder.' *Psychiatric Genetics 11*, 57–63.

Chapter 5

American Academy of Pediatrics (2001) 'The pediatrician's role in the diagnosis and management of autistic spectrum disorder in children.' *Pediatrics 107*, 1221–1226.

Chez, M.G., Chin, K., and Hung, P.C. (2004) 'Immunizations, immunology, and autism.' *Seminars in Pediatric Neurology 11*, 214–217.

Filipek, P.A., Accardo, P.J., Ashwal, S., *et al.* (2000) 'Practice parameter: Screening and diagnosis of autism.' Report of the Quality Standards Subcommittee of the American Academy of Neurology and Child Neurology Society. *Neurology 55*, 469–479.

Geschwind, D.H., Cummings, J.L., Hollander, E., *et al.* (1998) 'Autism screening and diagnosis: CAN consensus statement.' *CNS Spectrum 3*, 40–49.

Immunization Safety Review Committee, Board on Health Promotion and Disease Prevention, Institute of Medicine (2004) *Immunization Safety Review: Vaccines and Autism.* Washington, DC: National Academies Press.

Volkmar, F., Cook, E.H., Pomeroy, J., *et al.* (1999) 'Practice parameters for the assessment and treatment of children and adults with autism and other pervasive developmental disorders.' American Academy of Child and Adolescent Psychiatry Working Group on Quality Issues. *Journal of the American Academy of Child and Adolescent Psychiatry 38,* 32S–54S.

Chapter 6

Hyland, K. (2003) 'The lumbar puncture for diagnosis of pediatric neurotransmitter diseases.' *Annals of Neurology 54,* Suppl 6, S13–17.

Moretti, P., Sahoo, T., Hyland, K., *et al.* (2005) 'Cerebral folate deficiency with developmental delay, autism, and response to folinic acid.' *Neurology 64,* 1088–1090.

Pearl, P.L., Novotny, E.J., Acosta, M.T., *et al.* (2003) 'Succinic semialdehyde dehydrogenase deficiency in children and adults.' *Annals of Neurology 54,* Suppl 6, S73–S80.

Spence, S.J. (2004) 'The genetics of autism.' *Seminars in Pediatric Neurology 11,* 196–204.

Spence, S.J., Sharifi, P., and Wiznitzer, M. (2004) 'Autism spectrum disorder: Screening, diagnosis, and medical evaluation.' *Seminars in Pediatric Neurology 11,* 186–195.

Chapter 7

Bauman, M.L. and Kemper, T.L. (eds) (1994) *Neurobiology of Autism.* Baltimore, MD: Johns Hopkins University Press.

Bauman, M.L. and Kemper, T.L. (1986) 'Development of cerebellar abnormalities: A finding of early infantile autism.' *Neurology 36,* 190 (Abstract).

Chugani, D.C., Muzik, O., Behen, M., *et al.* (1999) 'Developmental changes in brain serotonin synthesis capacity in autistic and non-autistic children.' *Annals of Neurology 45,* 287–295.

Courchesne, E., Carper, R., and Akshoomoff, N. (2003) 'Evidence of brain overgrowth in the first year of life in autism.' *JAMA 290,* 3, 393–394.

Courchesne, E., Karns, C.M., Davis, H.R., *et al.* (2001) 'Unusual brain growth patterns in early life in patients with autistic disorder: An MRI study.' *Neurology 57,* 245–254.

Courchesne, E., Saitoh, O., Yeung-Courchesne, R., *et al.* (1994) 'Abnormality of cerebellar vermian lobules VI and VII in patients with infantile autism: Identification of hypoplastic and hyperplastic subgroups with MR imaging.' *American Journal of Roentgenology 162*, 123–130.

Dapretto, M., Davies, M.S., Pfeifer, J.H., *et al.* (2006) 'Understanding emotions in others: Mirror neuron dysfunction in children with autism spectrum disorders.' *Nature Neuroscience 9*, 1, 28–30.

Friedman, S.D., Shaw, D.W., Artu, A.A., *et al.* (2003) 'Regional brain chemical alterations in young children with autism spectrum disorder.' *Neurology 60*, 100–107.

Hardan, A.Y., Minshew, N.J., Mallikarjuhn, M., *et al.* (2001) 'Brain volume in autism.' *Journal of Child Neurology 16*, 421–424.

Hazlett, H.C., Poe, M.D., Gerig, G., *et al.* (2005). 'Cortical gray and white brain tissue volume in adolescents and adults with autism.' *Biological Psychiatry 59*, 1, 1–6.

Herbert, M.R., Harris, G.J., Adrien, K.T., *et al.* (2002) 'Abnormal asymmetry in language association cortex in autism.' *Annals of Neurology 52*, 588–596.

Herbert, M.R., Ziegler, D.A., Makris, N., *et al.* (2004) 'Localization of white matter volume increase in autism and developmental language disorder.' *Annals of Neurology 55*, 530–540.

Jones, C.R., Hansen, R., Krakowiak, P., *et al.* (2006) 'Autism and head circumference in the CHARGE study.' Presented at the IMFAR meeting in Montreal, Canada, June 1.

Just, M.A., Cherkassky, V.L., Keller, T.A., and Minshew, N.J. (2004) 'Cortical activation and synchronization during sentence comprehension in high functioning autism: Evidence of underconnectivity.' *Brain 127*, 8, 1811–1821.

Kaufmann, W.E., Cooper, K.L., Mostofsky, S.H., *et al.* (2003) 'Specificity of cerebellar vermian abnormalities in autism: A quantitative magnetic resonance imaging study.' *Journal of Child Neurology 18*, 463–470.

Koshino, H., Carpenter, P.A., Minshew, N.J., *et al.* (2005) 'Functional connectivity in fMRI working memory task in high-functioning autism.' *Neuroimage 24*, 810–821.

Lewine, J.D., Andrews, R., Chez, M.G., *et al.* (1999) 'Magnetoencephalographic patterns of epileptiform activity in children with regressive autism spectrum disorders.' *Pediatrics 104*, 405–418.

Muller, R.A., Cauich, C., Rubio, M.A., *et al.* (2004) 'Abnormal activity patterns in premotor cortex during sequence learning in autistic patients.' *Biological Psychiatry 56*, 5, 323–332.

Murphy, D.G.M., Critchley, H.D., Schmitz, N., *et al.* (2002) 'Asperger syndrome: A proton magnetic resonance spectroscopy study of the brain.' *Archives of General Psychiatry 59*, 885–891.

Neville, B.G. (1999) 'Magnetencephalographic patterns of epileptiform activity in children with regressive autism spectrum disorders.' *Pediatrics 103*, 55–58.

Raymond, G.V., Bauman, M.L., and Kemper, T.L. (1996) 'Hippocampus in autism: A Golgi analysis.' *Acta Neuropathologica (Berl) 91*, 117–119.

Sparks, B.F., Friedman, S.D., Shaw, D.W., *et al.* (2002) 'Brain structural abnormalities in young children with autism spectrum disorder.' *Neurology 59*, 184–192.

Vargas, D.L., Nascimbene, C., Krishnan, C., *et al.* (2005) 'Neuroglial activation and neuroinflammation in the brain of patients with autism.' *Annals of Neurology 57*, 67–81.

Chapter 8

EEG abnormalities and regression in ASD

Chez, M.G., Buchanan, T., Aimonovitch, M., *et al.* (2004) 'Frequency of EEG abnormalities in age matched siblings of autistic children with abnormal sleep EEG patterns.' *Epilepsy and Behavior 5*, 159–162.

Chez, M.G., Chang, M., Krasne, V., *et al.* (2006) 'Frequency of epileptiform EEG abnormalities in a sequential screening of autistic patients with no known clinical epilepsy from 1996–2005.' *Epilepsy and Behavior 8*, 267–271.

Chez, M.G., Buchanan, C., Zucker, M., and May, B. (1997) 'Value of 24 hour EEG versus routine EEG in detecting occult epileptic activity in children with pervasive developmental delays.' *Annals of Neurology 42*, 509 (Abstract).

Gubbay, S.S., Lobascher, M., and Kingerlee, P. (1970) 'A neurologic appraisal of autistic children: Results of a Western Australian survey.' *Developmental Medicine and Child Neurology 12*, 433–439.

Olsson, I., Steffenburg, S., and Gillberg, C. (1988) 'Epilepsy in autism and autistic-like conditions.' *Archives of Neurology 45*, 666–668.

Rapin, I. (1995) 'Autistic regression and disintegrative disorder: How important is the role of epilepsy?' *Seminars in Pediatric Neurology 2*, 4, 278–285.

Tuchman, R., and Jayakar, P., Yaylali, I., and Villalobos, R. (1998) 'Seizures and EEG findings in children with autism spectrum disorder.' *CNS Spectrums 3*, 3, 61–68.

Tuchman, R. and Rapin, I. (2002) 'Epilepsy in autism.' *The Lancet Neurology 1*, 352–358.

Landau-Kleffner syndrome and continuous spike-wave in sleep (LKS/CSWS) and neuroimaging studies in ASD and EEG abnormalities

Beaumanoir, A., Bureau, M., Deonna, T., Mira, L., and Tassinari, C.A. (eds) (1993) *Continuous Spikes and Waves During Slow Sleep Electrical Status Epilepticus During Slow Sleep: Acquired Epileptic Aphasia and Related Conditions.* Milan, Italy: Mariani Foundation.

Deonna, T. (1991) 'Acquired epileptiform aphasia in children (Landau-Kleffner syndrome).' *Journal of Clinical Neurophysiology 7,* 288–298.

Lewine, J.D., Andrews, R., Chez, M.G., *et al.* (1999) 'Magnetoencephalographic patterns of epileptiform activity in children with regressive autism spectrum disorders.' *Pediatrics 104,* 405–418.

Morrell, F.M., Whistler, W.W., Smith, M.C., *et al.* (1995) 'Landau-Kleffner syndrome: Treatment with subpial intracortical transaction.' *Brain 118,* 1529–1546.

Neville, B.G. (1999) 'Magnetoencephalographic patterns of epileptiform activity in children with regressive autism spectrum disorders.' *Pediatrics 103,* 55–58.

Treating interictal spikes on EEG: Cognitive effects of EEG abnormalities in the absence of seizures

Aldenkamp, A. and Arends, J. (2004) 'The relative influence of epileptic EEG discharges, short non-convulsive seizures, and type of epilepsy on cognitive function.' *Epilepsia 45,* 1, 54–65.

Deonna, T. (1995) 'Cognitive and behavioral disturbances as epileptic manifestations in children: An overview.' *Seminars in Pediatric Neurology 2,* 4, 254–260.

Perez, E.R. (1995) 'Syndromes of acquired epileptic aphasia and epilepsy with continuous spike-waves in sleep: Models for prolonged cognitive impairment of epileptic origin.' *Seminars in Pediatric Neurology 2,* 4, 269–277.

Pressler, R.M., Robinson, R.O., Wilson, G.A., and Binnie, C.D. (2005) 'Treatment of interictal epileptiform discharges can improve behavior in children with behavioral problems and epilepsy.' *Journal of Pediatrics 146,* 1, 112–117.

Immune abnormalities in epilepsy and autism

Pardo, C.A., Vargas, D.L., and Zimmerman, A. (2005) 'Immunity, neuroglia and neuroinflammation in autism.' *International Review of Psychiatry 17,* 6, 485–495.

Vargas, D.L., Nascimbene, C., Krishnan, C., Zimmerman, A.W., and Pardo, C.A. (2005) 'Neuroglial activation and neuroinflammation in the brain of patients with autism.' *Annals of Neurology 57,* 67–81.

Vezzani, A. (2006) 'Inflammation and epilepsy.' *Epilepsy Currents 5,* 1, 1–6.

Vezzani, A. and Granata, T. (2005) 'Brain inflammation in epilepsy: Experimental and clinical evidence.' *Epilepsia 46*, 11, 1724–1743.

Chapter 9

Cook, E.H. Jr. (2001) 'Genetics of autism.' *Journal of Child and Adolescent Psychiatric Clinics of North America 10*, 333–350.

Spence, S.J. (2004) 'Genetics of autism.' *Seminars in Pediatric Neurology 11*, 196–204.

Chapter 10

Baird, G., Simonoff, E., Pickles, A., *et al.* (2006) 'Prevalence of disorders of the autism spectrum in a population cohort of children in South Thames: The Special Needs and Autism Project (SNAP)' *The Lancet 368*, 210–215.

California Department of Developmental Services (2003) *Autistic Spectrum Disorders. Changes in the California Caseload. An Update: 1999 Through 2002.* Sacramento, CA: California Health and Human Services Agency.

Chakrabarti, S. and Fombonne, E. (2001) 'Pervasive developmental disorders in preschool children.' *JAMA 285*, 3093–3099.

Croen, L., Grether, J., Hoogstrate, J., and Selvin, S. (2002) 'The changing prevalence of autism in California.' *Journal of Autism and Developmental Disorders 32*, 3, 207–215.

Fombonne, E. (2001) 'Is there an epidemic of autism?' *Pediatrics 107*, 411– 413.

Gillberg, C., Cederlund, M., Lamberg, K., and Zeijlon, L. (2006) 'Brief report: "The autism epidemic": The registered prevalence of autism in a Swedish urban area.' *Journal of Autism and Developmental Disorders 36*, 429–435.

MIND Institute (2002) *Report to the Legislature on the Principal Findings from the Epidemiology of Autism in California.* Sacramento, CA: University of California, Davis.

Newschaffer, C.J., Falb, M.D., and Gurney, J.G. (2005) 'National autism prevalence trends from United States special education data.' *Pediatrics 115*, 3, e277–e282 (electronic article).

Shattuck, P.T. (2006) 'The contribution of diagnostic substitution to the growing administrative prevalence of autism in US special education.' *Pediatrics 117*, 4, 1028–1037.

Schieve, L.A., Rice, C., Boyle, C., Visser, S.N., Blumberg, S.J. (2006) 'Mental health in the United States: Parental report of diagnosed autism in children aged 4–17 years—United States, 2003–2004.' *Morbidity and Mortality Weekly Report 55*, 17, 481–486.

Yeargin-Alsip, M., Rice, C., Karapurkar, T., *et al.* (2003) 'Prevalence of autism in a US metropolitan area.' *JAMA 289*, 49–55.

Chapter 11
Immunization safety

Andrews, N., Miller, E., Taylor, B., *et al.* (2002) 'Recall bias, MMR, and autism.' *Archives of Diseases of Children 87*, 493–494.

Dales, L., Hammer, S.J., and Smith, N.J. (2001) 'Time trends in autism and MMR immunization coverage in California.' *JAMA 285*, 1183–1185.

Farrington, C.P., Miller, E., and Taylor, B. (2001) 'MMR and autism: Further evidence against a causal association.' *Vaccine 19*, 3632–3635.

Fombonne, E. and Chakrabarti, S. (2001) 'No evidence for a new variant of measles-mumps-rubella induced autism.' *Pediatrics 108*, E58.

Halsey, N.A., Hyman, S.L., and the conference writing panel (2001) 'Measles-mumps-rubella vaccine and autistic spectrum disorder.' Report from New Challenges in Childhood Immunizations Conference convened in Oak Brook, IL, June 11–12, 2000. *Pediatrics 107*, E84.

Hviid, A., Stellfeld, M., Wohlfahrt, J., *et al.* (2003) 'Association of thimerosal containing vaccine and autism.' *JAMA 290*, 1763–1766.

Immunization Safety Review Committee, Board on Health Promotion and Disease Prevention, Institute of Medicine (2004) *Immunization Safety Review: Vaccines and Autism.* Washington, DC: National Academies Press.

Kaye, J.A., del Mar Melero Montes, M., and Jick, H. (2001) 'Mumps, measles, and rubella vaccine and the incidence of autism recorded by general practitioners: A time trend analysis.' *British Medical Journal 322*, 460–463.

Madsen, K.M., Lauritsen, M.B., Pederson, C.B., *et al.* (2003) 'Thimerosal and the occurrence of autism: Negative ecological evidence from Danish population-based data.' *Pediatrics 112*, 604–606.

Takahashi, H., Suzumura, S., Shirakizawa, F., *et al.* (2003) 'An epidemiological study on Japanese autism concerning routine childhood immunization history.' *Japan Journal of Infectious Disease 56*, 114–117.

Environmental mercury risks and animal data

Hertz-Picciotto, I., Green, P.G., Croen, L., *et al.* (2006) 'Blood metal concentrations in the CHARGE study.' Presented first at IMFAR Meeting, Montreal, Canada, June 3.

Hornig, M., Chian, D., and Lipkin, W.I. (2004) 'Neurotoxic effects of postnatal thimerosal are mouse strain dependent.' *Molecular Psychiatry 9*, 833–845.

Institute for Vaccine Safety (2007) 'Thimerosal content in some currently manufactured U.S. licensed vaccines.' Table, available at www.vaccinesafety.edu/thi-table.htm (accessed November 2007).

Ip, P., Wong, V., Ho, M., *et al.* (2004) 'Mercury exposure in children with autistic spectrum disorder: case-control study.' *Journal of Child Neurology 19*, 6, 431–444.

Myers, G.J., Davidson, P.W., Cox, C., *et al.* (2003) 'Prenatal mercury exposure from ocean fish consumption in the Seychelles child development study.' *The Lancet 361*, 1686–1692.

Seidel, S., Kreutzer, R., Smith, D., *et al.* (2001) 'Assessment of commercial laboratories performing hair mineral analysis.' *JAMA 285*, 67–72.

Steindel, S.J., and Howanitz, P.J. (2001) 'The uncertainty of hair analysis for trace metals.' *JAMA 285*, 83–85.

Williams, P.G., Hersh, J., and Sears, L.L. (2006) 'A study of mercury levels in young children with autism using laboratory analysis of hair samples.' Presented first at IMFAR Meeting, Montreal, Canada, June 2.

MMR and autism

Murch, S.H. (2003) 'Separating inflammation from speculation in autism.' *The Lancet 362*, 14–98.

Murch, S.H., Anthony, A., Casson, D.H., *et al.* (2004) 'Retraction of an interpretation.' *The Lancet 363*, 750 [Commentary].

Wakefield, A.J., Murch, S.H., Anthony, A., *et al.* (1998) 'Ileal-lymphoid nodular hyperplasia, non-specific enteropathy, and pervasive developmental disorder of childhood.' *The Lancet 351*, 637–641.

Wakefield, A.J., Puleston, J.M., Montgomery, S.M., *et al.* (2000) 'The concept of entero-colonic encephalopathy, autism, and opioid receptor ligands.' *Alimentary Pharmacology and Therapeutics 16*, 663–674.

Chapter 12

Chez, M.G., Dowling, T., Patel, P., *et al.* (2007) 'Elevation of tumor necrosis factor-alpha in cerebrospinal fluid of autistic children.' *Pediatric Neurology 36*, 361–365.

Comi, A.M., Zimmerman, A.W., Frye, V.H., *et al.* (1999) 'Familial clustering of autoimmune disorders and evaluation of medical risk factors in autism.' *Journal of Child Neurology 14*, 388–394.

Connolly, A.M., Chez, M.G., Pestronk, A., *et al.* (1999) 'Serum antibodies to brain in Landau-Kleffner variant, autism, and other neurologic disorders.' *Journal of Pediatrics 134*, 607–613.

Connolly, A.M, Chez, M., Streif, E.M., *et al.* (2006) 'Brain-derived neurotrophic factor and autoantibodies to neural antigens in sera of children with autistic spectrum disorders, Landau-Kleffner syndrome, and epilepsy.' *Biological Psychiatry 59*, 354–363.

Gupta, S. (2000) 'Immunological treatments for autism.' *Journal of Autism and Developmental Disorders 30*, 475–479.

Gupta, S., Aggarwal, S., and Heads, C. (1996) 'Brief report. Dysregulated immune system in children with autism: Beneficial effects of intravenous immune globulin on autistic characteristics.' *Journal of Autism and Developmental Disorders 26*, 439–452.

Nelson, K.B., Grether, J.K., Croen, L.A., *et al.* (2001) 'Neuropeptides and neurotrophins in neonatal blood of children with autism and mental retardation.' *Annals of Neurology 49*, 597–606.

Pardo, C., Vargas, D.L., and Zimmerman, A.W. (2005) 'Immunity, neuroglia, and neuroinflammation in autism.' *International Review of Psychiatry 17*, 485–486.

Vargas, D.L., Nascimbene, C., Krishnan, C., *et al.* (2005) 'Neuroglial activation and neuroinflammation in the brain of patients with autism.' *Annals of Neurology 57*, 67–81.

Vezzani, A. (2005) 'Inflammation and epilepsy.' *Epilepsy Currents 5*, 1, 1–6.

Vezzani, A. and Granata, T. (2005) 'Brain inflammation in epilepsy: Experimental and clinical evidence.' *Epilepsia 46*, 11, 1724–1743.

Warren, R.P., Margaretten, N.C., Pace, N.C., *et al.* (1986) 'Immune abnormalities in patients with autism.' *Autism and Developmental Disorders 16*, 139.

Chapter 13

No references.

Chapter 14

Carmel, R., Melnyk, S., and James, S.J. (2003) 'Cobalamin deficiency with and without neurologic abnormalities: Differences in homocysteine and methionine metabolism.' *Blood 101*, 8, 3302–3308.

James, S.J., Cutler, P., Melnyk, S., *et al.* (2004) 'Metabolic markers of increased oxidative stress and impaired methylation capacity of children with autism.' *American Journal of Clinical Nutrition 80*, 6, 1611–1617.

James, S.J., Slikker, W. 3rd, Melnyk, S., *et al.* (2005) 'Thimerosal neurotoxicity is associated with glutathione depletion: Protection with glutathione precursors.' *Neurotoxicology 26*, 1, 1–8.

Chapters 15 and 16

No references.

Chapter 17

Steindal, S.J. and Howanitz, P.J. (2001) 'The uncertainty of hair analysis for trace metals.' *JAMA, 285*, 83–85.

Seidel, S., Kreutzer, R., Smith, D., McNeel, S., and Gillis, D. (2001) 'Assessment of commercial laboratories performing hair mineral analysis.' *JAMA, 285*, 67–72.

Hertz-Picciotto, I., Croen, L., Hansen, R., Jones, C.R., van de Water, J., and Pessah, I.N. (2006) 'Assessment of environmental and genetic risk factors in children with autism.' *Environ. Health Perspective 114(7)*, 1119–1125.

Schechter, R. and Grether, J.K. (2008) 'Continuing increases in autism reported to California's developmental services system.' *Archives of General Psychiatry 65(1)*, 19–24.

Chapter 18

No references.

Chapter 19

Aman, M.G. and Madrid, A. (1999) 'Atypical antipsychotics in persons with developmental disabilities.' *Mental Retardation Developmental Disabilities Research Review 5*, 253–263.

Campbell, M., Anderson, L.T., Meier, M., *et al.* (1978) 'A comparison of haloperidol and behavioral therapy and their interaction in autistic children.' *Journal of the American Academy of Child Psychiatry 17*, 640–655.

Gagliano, A., Germano, E., Pustorino, G., *et al.* (2004) 'Risperidone treatment of children with autistic disorder: effectiveness, tolerability, and pharmacokinetic implications.' *Journal of Child and Adolescent Psychopharmacology 14*, 39–47.

Locascio, J.J., Malone, R.P., Small, A.M., *et al.* (1991) 'Factors related to haloperidol response and dyskinesias in autistic children.' *Psychopharmacology Bulletin 27*, 119–126.

Malone, R.P., Cater, J., Sheikh, R.M., *et al.* (2001) 'Olanzipine versus haloperidol in children with autistic disorder.' *Journal of the American Academy of Child and Adolescent Psychiatry 40*, 8, 887–894.

Malone, R.P., Ernst, M., Godfrey, K.A., *et al.* (1991) 'Repeated episodes of neuroleptic-related dyskinesias in autistic children.' *Psychopharmacology Bulletin 27*, 113–117.

Mandoki, M.W. (1995) 'Risperidone treatment of children and adolescents: Increased risk of extrapyramidal side effects?' *Journal of Child and Adolescent Psychopharmacology 5*, 49–67.

Martin, A., Koenig, K., Scahill, L., *et al.* (1999) 'Open-label quetiapine in the treatment of children and adolescents with autistic disorder.' *Journal of Child and Adolescent Psychopharmacology 9*, 99–107.

Martin, A., Scahill, L., Anderson, G.M., *et al.* (2004) 'Weight and leptin changes among risperidone-treated youths with autism: 6-month prospective data.' *American Journal of Psychiatry 161*, 1125–1127.

McDougle, C.J., Kem, D.L., and Posey, D.J. (2002) 'Case series: Use of ziprasidone for maladaptive symptoms in youths with autism.' *Journal of the American Academy of Child and Adolescent Psychiatry 41*, 8, 921–927.

McDougle, C.J., Stigler, K.A., and Posey, D.J. (2003) 'Treatment of aggression in children with autism and conduct disorder.' *Journal of Clinical Psychiatry 64*, 16–25.

Research Units on Pediatric Psychopharmacology Autism Network (2002) 'A double blind, placebo controlled trial of risperidone in children with autistic disorder.' *New England Journal of Medicine 347*, 314–321.

Silva, R.R., Malone, R.P., Anderson, L.T., *et al.* (1993) 'Haloperidol withdrawal and weight changes in autistic children.' *Psychopharmacology Bulletin 29*, 287–291.

Stigler, K.A., Posey, D.J., and McDougle, C.J. (2004) 'Aripiprazole for maladaptive behavior in pervasive developmental disorders.' *Journal of Child and Adolescent Psychiatry 14*, 3, 455–463.

Zuddas, A., Ledda, M.G., Fratta, A., *et al.* (1996) 'Clinical effects of clozapine on autistic disorder.' *American Journal of Psychiatry 153*, 5, 738.

Antidepressant medications in autism

Aman, M.G., Arnold, L.E., and Armstrong, S.C. (1999) 'Review of serotonergic agents and pervasive behaviors in patients with developmental disabilities.' *Mental Retardation and Developmental Disability Research Review 5*, 279–289.

Chugani, D.C. (2002) 'Role of altered brain serotonin mechanisms in autism.' *Molecular Psychiatry 7*, Suppl 2, S16–S17.

Cook, E.H., Rowlett, R., Jaselskis, C., *et al.* (1992) 'Fluoxetine treatment of children and adults with autistic disorder and mental retardation.' *Journal of the American Academy of Child and Adolescent Psychiatry 31*, 739–745.

Delong, G.R., Ritch, C.R., and Burch, S. (2002) 'Fluoxetine response in children with autistic spectrum disorders: Correlation with familial major affective disorder and intellectual achievement.' *Developmental Medicine and Child Neurology 44*, 652–659.

Delong, G.R., Teague, L.A., and McSwain-Kamran, M. (1998) 'Effects of fluoxetine treatment in young children with idiopathic autism.' *Developmental Medicine and Child Neurology 40*, 551–562.

Fatemi, S.H., Realmuto, G.M., Khan, L., *et al.* (1998) 'Fluoxetine treatment of adolescent patients with autism: A longitudinal open trial.' *Journal of Autism and Developmental Disorders 28*, 303–307.

Gordon, C.T., State, R.C., Nelson, C., *et al.* (1993) 'A double-blind comparison of clomipramine, desipramine, and placebo in the treatment of autistic disorder.' *Archives of General Psychiatry 50*, 441–447.

McDougle, C.J., Brodkin, E.S., Naylor, S.T., *et al.* (1998) 'Sertraline in adults with pervasive developmental disorders: A prospective open label investigation.' *Journal of Clinical Psychopharmacology 18*, 62–66.

McDougle, C.J., Kresch, L.E., and Posey, D.J. (2000) 'Repetitive thoughts and behavior in pervasive developmental disorders: Treatment with serotonin reuptake inhibitors.' *Journal of Autism and Developmental Disorders 30*, 427–435.

Remington, G., Sloman, L., Konstantareas, M., *et al.* (2001) 'Clomipramine versus haloperidol in the treatment of autistic disorder: A double-blind, placebo-controlled crossover study.' *Journal of Clinical Psychopharmacology 21*, 440–444.

Steingard, R.J., Zimnitzky, B., DeMaso, D.R., *et al.* (1997) 'Sertraline treatment of transition-associated anxiety and agitation in children with autistic disorder.' *Journal of Child and Adolescent Psychopharmacology 7*, 9–15.

Strauss, W.L., Unis, A.S., Cowan, C., *et al.* (2002) 'Fluorine magnetic resonance spectroscopy measurement of brain fluvoxamine and fluoxetine in pediatric patients treated for pervasive developmental disorders.' *American Journal of Psychiatry 159*, 755–760.

Attention deficit disorder in ASD

Aman, M.G. (1996) 'Stimulant drugs in the developmental disabilities revisited.' *Journal of Developmental and Physical Disabilities 8*, 347–365.

Aman, M.G. and Langworthy, K.S. (2000) 'Pharmacotherapy for hyperactivity in children with autism and other pervasive developmental disorders.' *Journal of Autism and Developmental Disorders 30*, 451–459.

Chez, M.G., Becker, M., Kessler, J., *et al.* (2003) 'Psychostimulant use in children with autistic spectrum disorder.' *Annals of Neurology 54*, Suppl 7, 147 (Abstract).

Frankenhauser, M.P., Karumanchi, V.C., German, M.L., *et al.* (1992) 'A double-blind placebo-controlled study of the efficacy of transdermal clonidine in autism.' *Journal of Clinical Psychiatry 53*, 77–82.

Handen, B.L., Johnson, C.R., and Lubetsky, M. (2000) 'Efficacy of methylphenidate among children with autism and symptoms of attention-deficit hyperactivity disorder.' *Journal of Autism and Developmental Disorders 30*, 245–255.

Jaselskis, C.A., Cook, E.H., Fletcher, K.E., *et al.* (1992) 'Clonidine treatment of hyperactive and impulsive children with autistic disorder.' *Journal of Clinical Psychopharmacology 12*, 322–327.

Posey, D., Puntney, J., Sasher, T., *et al.* (2004) 'Guanfacine treatment of hyperactivity and inattention in autism: A retrospective analysis of 80 cases.' *Journal of Child Adolescent Psychopharmacology 14*, 233–241.

Stingler, K., Desmond, L., Posey, D., *et al.* (2004) 'A naturalistic retrospective analysis of psychostimulants in pervasive developmental disorders.' *Journal of Child and Adolescent Psychopharmacology 14*, 49–56.

Mood-stabilizing medications

Belsito, K.M., Law, P.A., Kirk, K.S., *et al.* (2001) 'Lamotrigine therapy for autistic disorder: A randomized double-blind, placebo-controlled study.' *Journal of Autism and Developmental Disorders 31*, 2, 175–181.

Chez, M.G., Memon, S., and Hung, P.C. (2004) 'Neurological treatment strategies in autism: An overview of medical intervention strategies.' *Seminars in Pediatric Neurology 11*, 229–235.

Hollander, E., Dolgoff-Kaspar, R., Cartwright, C., *et al.* (2001) 'An open trial of divalproex sodium in autistic spectrum disorders.' *Journal of Clinical Psychiatry 62*, 530–534.

Self-injury/aggression

Campbell, M., Anderson, L.T., Small, A.M., *et al.* (1993) 'Naltrexone in autistic children: Behavioral symptoms and attentional learning.' *Journal of the American Academy of Child and Adolescent Psychiatry 32*, 1283–1291.

Fraser, W.I., Ruedrich, S., Kerr, M., *et al,* (1998) 'Beta-adrenergic blockers.' In S. Reiss and M.G. Aman (eds) *Psychiatric Medications and Developmental Disabilities: The International Consensus Handbook* (pp.271–290). Columbus, OH: Ohio State University, Nissonger Center.

Feldman, H.M., Kolmen, V.C., and Gonzaga, A.M. (1999) 'Naltrexone and communication skills in young children with autism.' *Journal of the American Academy of Child and Adolescent Psychiatry 38*, 587–593.

McDougle, C.J., Stigler, K.A., and Posey, D.J. (2003) 'Treatment of aggression in children with autism and conduct disorder.' *Journal of Clinical Psychiatry 64*, Suppl 4, 16–25.

Willemsen-Swinkels, S.H., Buitelaar, J.K., Nihof, G.J., *et al.* (1995) 'Failure of naltrexone hydrochloride to reduce self-injurious and autistic behavior in mentally retarded adults: Double-blind placebo-controlled studies.' *Archives of General Psychiatry 52*, 766–773.

Willemsen-Swinkels, S.H., Buitelaar, J.K., and van Engeland, H. (1996) 'The effects of chronic naltrexone treatment in young autistic children: A double-blind, placebo-controlled crossover study.' *Biological Psychiatry 39*, 1023–1031.

Zingarelli, G., Ellman, G., Hom, A., *et al.* (1992) 'Clinical effects of naltrexone on autistic behavior.' *American Journal of Mental Retardation 97*, 57–63.

Chapter 20

Besag, F.M.C. (1995) 'The therapeutic dilemma: Treating subtle seizures or indulging in electroencephalogram cosmetics.' *Seminars in Pediatric Neurology 2*, 261–268.

Kanner, A.M. (2000) 'The treatment of seizure disorders and EEG abnormalities in children with autistic spectrum disorders: Are we getting ahead of ourselves?' *Journal of Autism and Developmental Disorders 30*, 491–495.

Tuchman, R. (2000) 'Treatment of seizure disorders and EEG abnormalities in children with autism spectrum disorders.' *Journal of Autism and Developmental Disorders 30*, 485–489.

Treatment with valproic acid in autism with abnormal EEG, and other anticonvulsant use in autism for behavior

Bardenstein, R., Chez, M.G., Helfand, B.T., *et al.* (1998) 'Improvement in EEG and clinical function in pervasive developmental delay (PDD): Effect of valproic acid.' *Neurology 50*, Suppl 4, A86 (Abstract).

Belsito, K.M., Law, P.A., Kirk, K.S., *et al.* (2001) 'Lamotrigine therapy for autistic disorder: A randomized double-blind, placebo-controlled study.' *Journal of Autism and Developmental Disorders 31*, 2, 175–181.

Chez, M.G., Buchanan, C., Loeffel, M., *et al.* (1998) 'Treatment of electroencephalographic epileptiform activity on overnight EEG studies in children with pervasive developmental disorder or autism: Defining similarities to the Landau-Kleffner syndrome.' *Journal of Developmental Learning Disorders 2*, 217–229.

Chez, M.G., Chang, M., Krasne, V., *et al.* (2006) 'Frequency of epileptiform EEG abnormalities in a sequential screening of autistic patients with no known clinical epilepsy from 1996–2005.' *Epilepsy and Behavior 8*, 267–271.

Deonna, T., Ziegler, A., Maeder, M., *et al.* (1995) 'Reversible behavioral autistic-like regression: A manifestation of a special (new?) epileptic syndrome in a 28-month-old child. A 2-year longitudinal study.' *Neurocase 1*, 91–95.

Hollander, E., Dolgoff-Kaspar, R., Cartwright, C., *et al.* (2001) 'An open trial of divalproex sodium in autistic spectrum disorders.' *Journal of Clinical Psychiatry 62*, 530–534.

Plioplys, A.V. (1994) 'Autism: Electroencephalogram abnormalities and clinical improvement with valproic acid.' *Archives of Pediatric and Adolescent Medicine 148*, 220–222.

Treatment with corticosteroids

Aykut-Bingol, C., Arman, A., Tokol, O., *et al.* (1998) 'Pulse methylprednisolone therapy in Landau-Kleffner syndrome.' *Journal of Epilepsy 9*, 189–191.

Chez, M.G., Buchanan, C, Loeffel, M.F., *et al.* (1998) 'Practical treatment with pulse-dose corticosteroids in pervasive developmental disorder or autistic patients with abnormal sleep EEG and language delay.' In M. Perat (ed) *New Developments in Child Neurology* (pp.695–698). Bologna, Italy: Monduzzi Editore.

Chez, M.G., Loeffel, M., Buchanan, C., *et al.* (1998) 'Pulse high-dose steroids as combination therapy with valproic acid in epileptic aphasia patients with pervasive developmental delay or autism.' *Annals of Neurology 44*, 539 (Abstract).

Marescaux, C., Hirsch, E., Finck, S., *et al.* (1990) 'Landau-Kleffner syndrome: A pharmacologic study of five cases.' *Epilepsia 31*, 768–777.

Stefanotos, G.A., Grover, W., and Geller, E. (1995) 'Case study: Corticosteroid treatment of language regression in pervasive developmental disorder.' *Journal of the American Academy of Child and Adolescent Psychiatry 34*, 8, 1107–1111.

Trauner, D.A., Nabangchang, C., Ballantyne, A., *et al.* (2002) 'Developmental aphasia with epileptiform abnormalities on EEG: Clinical features and response to prednisone.' *Annals of Neurology 52*, 3, S66–67 (Abstract).

Treatment with subpial surgery

Lewine, J.D., Andrews, R., Chez, M.G., *et al.* (1999) 'Magnetoencephalographic patterns of epileptiform activity in children with regressive autism spectrum disorders.' *Pediatrics 104*, 405–418.

Nass, R., Gross, A., Wisoff, J., *et al.* (1999) 'Outcome of multiple subpial transaction for autistic epileptiform regression.' *Pediatric Neurology 21*, 464–470.

Neville, B.G., Harkness, W.F., Cross, J.H., *et al.* (1997) 'Surgical treatment of severe autistic regression in childhood epilepsy.' *Pediatric Neurology 16*, 137–140.

Chapter 21
Immunoglobulin therapy

Gupta, S. (1999) 'Treatment of children with autism with intravenous immunoglobulin.' *Journal of Child Neurology 14*, 203–205.

Gupta, S. (2000). 'Immunological treatments for autism.' *Journal of Autism and Developmental Disorders 30*, 475–479.

Gupta, S., Aggarwal, S., and Heads, C. (1996) 'Brief report. Dysregulated immune system in children with autism: Beneficial effects of intravenous immune globulin on autistic characteristics.' *Journal of Autism and Developmental Disorders 26*, 439–452.

Plioplys, A.V. (2000) 'Intravenous immunoglobulin treatment in autism.' *Journal of Autism and Developmental Disorders 30*, 73–74.

Corticosteroids

Aykut-Bingol, C., Arman, A., Tokol, O., *et al.* (1998) 'Pulse methylprednisolone therapy in Landau-Kleffner syndrome.' *Journal of Epilepsy 9*, 189–191.

Chez, M.G., Buchanan, C, Loeffel, M.F., *et al.* (1998) 'Practical treatment with pulse-dose corticosteroids in pervasive developmental disorder or autistic patients with abnormal sleep EEG and language delay.' In M. Perat (ed) *New Developments in Child Neurology* (pp.695–698). Bologna, Italy: Monduzzi Editore.

Marescaux, C., Hirsch, E., Finck, S., *et al.* (1990) 'Landau-Kleffner syndrome: A pharmacologic study of five cases.' *Epilepsia 31*, 768–777.

Stefanotos, G.A., Grover, W., and Geller, E. (1995) 'Case study: Corticosteroid treatment of language regression in pervasive developmental disorder.' *Journal of the American Academy of Child and Adolescent Psychiatry 34*, 8, 1107–1111.

Trauner, D.A., Nabangchang, C., Ballantyne, A., *et al.* (2002) 'Developmental aphasia with epileptiform abnormalities on EEG: Clinical features and response to prednisone.' *Annals of Neurology 52*, 3, S66–67 (Abstract).

Chapter 22
Secretin

Chez, M.G., Buchanan, C.P., Bagan, B.T., *et al.* (2000) 'Secretin and autism: A two-part clinical investigation.' *Journal of Autism and Developmental Disorders 30*, 87–94.

Dunn-Geier, J., Ho, H.H., Auersperg, E., *et al.* (2000) 'Effect of secretin on children with autism: A randomized controlled trial.' *Developmental Medicine and Child Neurology 42*, 796–802.

Horvath, K. and Perman, J.A. (2002) 'Autism and gastrointestinal symptoms.' *Current Gastrointestinal Report 4*, 251–258.

Sandler, A.D. and Bodfish, J.W. (2000) 'Placebo effects in autism: Lessons from secretin.' *Journal of Developmental and Behavioral Pediatrics 21*, 347–350.

Sponheim, E., Oftedal, G., and Helverschou, S.B. (2002) 'Multiple doses of secretin in the treatment of autism: A controlled study.' *Acta Paediatrica 91*, 540–545.

Unis, A.S., Munson, J.A., Rogers, S.J., *et al.* (2002) 'A randomized, double-blind, placebo-controlled trial of porcine versus synthetic secretin for reducing symptoms of autism.' *Journal of the American Academy of Child and Adolescent Psychiatry 41*, 1315–1321.

Gluten/casein-free diet

Cornish, E. (2002) 'Gluten and casein free diets in autism: A study of the effects on food choice and nutrition.' *Journal of Human Nutrition and Diet 15*, 261–269.

Sponheim, E. (1991) ['Gluten-free diet in infantile autism: A therapeutic trial.'] Article in Norwegian. *Tidsskreport for Den Norske Laegeforen 111*, 704–707.

Bacterial overgrowth theory

Sandler, R.H., Finegold, S.M., Bolte, E.R., *et al.* (2000) 'Short-term benefit from oral vancomycin treatment of regressive-onset autism.' *Journal of Child Neurology 15*, 429–435.

Encopresis

Chez, M.G., Nowinski, C.V., and Buchanan, C.P. (2000) 'Presence of gastrointestinal symptoms in children with primary diagnoses of autistic disorders.' *Annals of Neurology 48*, 3, 542 (Abstract).

Chapter 23
Valproic acid/steroid therapy/EEG treatment

Bardenstein, R., Chez, M.G., Helfand, B.T., *et al.* (1998) 'Improvement in EEG and clinical function in pervasive developmental delay (PDD): Effect of valproic acid.' *Neurology 50*, Suppl 4, A86 (Abstract).

Buitelaar, J.K., van Engeland, H., de Kogel, K.H., *et al.* (1992) 'The use of adrenocorticotrophic hormone (4-9) analog ORG 2766 in autistic children: Effects on the organization of behavior.' *Biological Psychiatry 311*, 1119–1129.

Chez, M.G., Buchanan, C., Loeffel, M.F., *et al.* (1998) 'Practical treatment with pulse-dose corticosteroids in pervasive developmental disorder or autistic patients with abnormal sleep EEG and language delay.' In M. Perat (ed) *New Developments in Child Neurology* (pp.695–698). Bologna, Italy: Monduzzi Editore.

Chez, M.G., Loeffel, M., Buchanan, C., *et al.* (1998) 'Pulse high-dose steroids as combination therapy with valproic acid in epileptic aphasia patients with pervasive developmental delay or autism.' *Annals of Neurology 44*, 539 (Abstract).

Hollander, E., Dolgoff-Kaspar, R., Cartwright, C., *et al.* (2001). 'An open trial of divalproex sodium in autistic spectrum disorders.' *Journal of Clinical Psychiatry 62*, 530–534.

Levisohn, P.M. (2004) 'Electroencephalography findings in autism: Similarities and differences from Landau-Kleffner syndrome.' *Seminars in Pediatric Neurology 11*, 218–224.

Plioplys, A.V. (1994) 'Autism: Electroencephalogram abnormalities and clinical improvement with valproic acid.' *Archives of Pediatric and Adolescent Medicine 148*, 220–222.

Stefanotos, G.A., Grover, W., and Geller, E. (1995) 'Case study: Corticosteroid treatment of language regression in pervasive developmental disorder.' *Journal of the American Academy of Child and Adolescent Psychiatry 34*, 8, 1107–1111.

Trauner, D.A., Nabangchang, C., Ballantyne, A., *et al.* (2002) 'Developmental aphasia with epileptiform abnormalities on EEG: Clinical features and response to prednisone.' *Annals of Neurology 52*, 3, S66–67 (Abstract).

Tuchman, R. (2000) 'Treatment of seizure disorders and EEG abnormalities in children with autism spectrum disorders.' *Journal of Autism and Developmental Disorders 30*, 485–489.

Cholinergic receptors and cholinesterase inhibitors

Chez, M.G., Aimonovitch, M., Buchanan, T., *et al.* (2007) 'Treating autistic spectrum disorders in children: Utility of the cholinesterase inhibitor rivastigmine tartrate.' *Journal of Child Neurology 19*, 165–169.

Chez, M.G., Buchanan, T., Becker, M., *et al.* (2003) 'Donezepil hydrochloride: A double-blind study in autistic children.' *Journal of Pediatric Neurology 1*, 83–88.

Hardan, A.Y. and Handen, B.L. (2002) 'A retrospective open trial of adjunctive donepezil in children and adolescents with autistic disorder.' *Journal of Child and Adolescent Psychopharmacology 12*, 237–241.

Hertzman, M. (2003) 'Galantamine in the treatment of adult autism: A report of three clinical cases.' *International Journal of Psychiatry and Medicine 33*, 395–398.

Perry, E.K., Lee, M.L., Martin-Ruiz, C.M., *et al.* (2001) 'Cholinergic activity in autism: Abnormalities in the cerebral cortex and basal forebrain.' *American Journal of Psychiatry 158*, 1058–1066.

Glutamate/memantine

Chez, M.G., Burton, Q., Dowling, T., *et al.* (in press) 'Memantine as adjunctive therapy in children diagnosed with autistic spectrum disorders: An observation of initial clinical response and maintenance tolerability.' *Journal of Child Neurology 22*, 5, 574–579.

Chez, M.G., Hung, P.C., Chin, K., *et al.* (2004) 'Memantine experience in children and adolescents with autistic spectrum disorders.' *Annals of Neurology 56*, 8, S109 (Abstract).

Owley, T., Salt, J., Guter, S., *et al.* (2006) 'A prospective, open-label trial of memantine in the treatment of cognitive, behavioral, and memory dysfunction in pervasive developmental disorders.' *Journal of Child and Adolescent Psychopharmacology 16*, 5, 517–524.

Purcell, A.E., Jeon, O.H., Zimmerman, A.W., *et al.* (2001) 'Postmortem brain abnormalities of the glutamate neurotransmitter system in autism.' *Neurology 57*, 1618–1628.

Natural supplements

Chez, M.G., Buchanan, C., Aimonovitch, M.C., *et al.* (2002) 'Double blind placebo-controlled study of L-carnosine in children with autistic spectrum disorders.' *Journal of Child Neurology 17*, 833–837.

Appendix 2

Glossary

Acetylcholinesterase inhibitor: Drugs that increase acetyl choline loss by inhibiting metabolism of that chemical in the brain.

Acetyl choline: Chemical that acts a neurotransmitter in the brain and may affect frontal lobe and nicotinic receptors in autism.

Alpha adrenergic: Drugs that block adrenergic excess or fight or flight; these are alpha adrenergic blockers like clonidine, etc.

Alternative practice: Treatment that lies outside of scientific avenues of medicine, usually non-proven therapy.

Ambulatory EEG: A form of EEG that can be worn while a patient moves around doing normal activity.

Amino acids: Protein building blocks that can cause disease if abnormally metabolized, such as in PKU (phenylketonuria).

Angelman syndrome: Genetic disorder on chromosome 15 also known as Happy Puppet Syndrome. This is usually associated with more severe epilepsy, abnormal EEG, and mental retardation and aphasia of speech. Typical dysmorphic appearance includes type of face with peg like teeth, and puppet-like features.

Anterior cingulate gyrus: Section running above the corpus callosum or middle connecting parts of the two halves of the brain, important for attention and interconnecting the two halves of the brain.

Anticonvulsants: Drugs that stop seizures or convulsions. Also known as anti-epileptic drugs. Types of anticonvulsants include Trileptol (oxcarbazepine), Tegretol (carbamezepine), Lamictal (lamotrigine), Keppra (levetiracetam), Dilantin (phenytoin), phenobarbitol, Depakote (valproic acid), Zonegran (zonisamide), Zarontin (ethoxsuccimide), and Felbatol (felbamate).

Antidepressants: Medications that are used to treat depression. Can include tricyclic, monoamine oxidase inhibitors, and serotonin reuptake inhibitors, and mixed types.

Antipsychotic medications: Drugs typically used for psychosis or schizophrenia; there are also now more modern versions called atypical antipsychotics. These typically inhibit various dopamine receptors in the brain. Older typical drugs include Haldol (haloperidol), Mellaril (thioridazine), and Thorazine (chlorpromazine). Newer atypical antipsychotic medications include Risperdal (risperidone), Zyprexa (olanzapine), Seroquel (quetiapine), Geodon (ziprasidone), Abilify (aripiprazole), and Clozaril (clozapine).

Applied behavioral analysis (ABA): An intensive educational behavioral therapy, or Lovaas Therapy (named after the initiator Dr. Ivan Lovaas). The therapy consists of repeated "discreet learning trials" or repetitive teaching of rote activities, using a reward system to teach desired behaviors.

Aricept: Trade name for donezepil, a type of cholinesterase inhibitor drug usually used in Alzheimer's disease.

ARX-gene: A recently discovered gene associated with seizures and X-linked retardation, usually in boys.

Asperger's syndrome: Form of high-functioning autism that may have superior or normal IQ, later diagnosis, and have more fluent language. May be subtle in differences from high-functioning autism in degree of certain auditory processing issues, spelling, and less problem with background stimulation. Classic narrow interests.

Astrocyte: Type of glial cell.

Autism: Specific behavioral disorder of childhood with lack of normal speech and communication, social, and emotional development with onset in the first 24 months of life.

Autosomal dominant: Gene type that needs to be inherited from only one parent from a cellular non-sex chromosome to cause a genetic effect.

Autosomal recessive: Gene type that needs to be inherited from both parents to cause an effect.

Autistic spectrum disorder (ASD): A group of conditions that have features of autism including secondary autism, Rett's syndrome, Asperger's, and PDD-NOS.

Batten's disease: An inherited genetic disease with abnormal development or regression in childhood and also called neuronal ceroid lipofuscinosis (NCL). Can mimic autistic regression clinically.

Behavioral therapy: Repetitive behavioral technique to obtain desired behavior and discourage unwanted behaviors. Different types include modifying autism with repetitive activity.

Bipolar disorder/manic-depression: Psychiatric condition with mood swings based on presumed biochemical imbalance within the limbic system. Families with this have been highly associated with more autism in family members. Treatment is with mood-stabilizing drugs and atypical antipsychotics.

Blood-brain barrier: Tissue surrounding the brain that isolates and separates the blood and peripheral immune system from the brain immune and circulatory system. Consists of the glial membrane surfaces, the dura, pia, and arachnoid matter.

Brain-derived neurotrophic factor (BDNF): A neuronal growth stimulant that may be produced as a result of stress to the nervous system, or may be needed to prevent impairment to the nervous system. May be impaired in Rett's syndrome.

Broca's area: Part of the brain involved in expressive speech, localized to inferior and posterior portion of the left frontal lobe of the brain in most people.

CAN (Cure Autism Now): Charity supporting mainstream genetic and scientific research in autism. This group recently merged with Autism Speaks. (See also Appendix 3: Resources.)

Cerebellum: Posterior primitive brain structure that coordinates balance and movement, but also plays a role in speech and learning. May be smaller or damaged according to some theories and research in autism. The vermis is the middle structure of the cerebellum. Purkinje cells are organizing cells important for learning and are damaged or lost due to inflammation or other causes in some autism research findings.

Chelation: Treatment that binds positive metal ions with agents that chemically help remove them from tissues in the body. These drugs may also bond important useful metals or positive ions such as calcium and iron.

Childhood disintegrative disorder: Late onset of loss of language and social skills often for no identifiable reason with loss of social interaction and language after age three to four years or later with no identifiable degenerative known disease or reason. Also in the DSM as part of the autistic disorders.

Cholinesterase inhibitor: Similar to acetylcholinesterase inhibitor but is a more generic cholinesterase inhibitor in addition to an acetyl cholinesterase inhibitor.

Chromosome: Unit of genetic material that help make up a cell's genetic stored material. A cell can have many chromosomes, and different species may have different numbers of chromosomes. Humans have 46 cellular chromosomes, including two sex chromosomes XX (female) or XY (male).

CSF (cerebrospinal fluid): Fluid surrounding the brain, usually clear; may contain markers of inflammation or chemical activity of the brain if studied.

CSF neurotransmitter deficiency: This is a rare set of conditions that have been associated with PDD and types of autism where folinic acid or certain monoamine precursors are low in children with global delay, seizures, or degeneration.

Cytokine: Proteins produced to react to inflammation and foreign stimuli by the immune system, produced by neuroglial cells in the brain.

DAN (Defeat Autism Now): Group associated with the Autism Research Review International and founded by Dr. Bernard Rimland.

Deletion: Absences of part of the genetic material from a piece of a chromosome.

Depakote/Depakene (valproic acid): A type of anti-epileptic drug that can change EEGs and increase the GABA effect.

Digital EEG: Electrical technique measures digital vs. analog data collection for brain electrical activity. Can be regular or ambulatory. Most EEG today is collected in digital format.

DNA (deoxynucleic acid): Raw material that makes the building blocks of genetic matter in the cell nucleus.

Dopamine: A monoaminergic neurotransmitter that in excess causes tics, mania, psychosis, and lack of which may affect attention, and moods. Blocked by atypical and typical antipsychotics.

Double-blind study: The patient and the treating doctor do not know for sure which drug or placebo a patient is taking, so results are not biased by expectations.

EEG (Electroencephalogram): A technique that measures brain electrical activity. It looks for slow or abnormally excitable changes that can detect epilepsy for example.

Floortime: Behavioral method therapy of Dr. Stanley Greenspan utilizing modeling of social and play behaviors.

Fragile X: A genetic syndrome in males that may mimic some autistic features in global delay, but also rarely in females with mosaicism. Associated with mental retardation, sterility, low set ears, large testicles at puberty, hypotonia, and severe hyperactivity usually. Genetic testing is available.

Frontal lobes: Anterior portion of the cerebral hemisphere of the brain; control higher functions of executive decision making in humans.

GABA (Gamma-aminobutyric acid): An inhibitory amino acid neurotransmitter in the central nervous system.

Genome: Refers to entire collection of genetic material in a species, e.g. the human genome has recently been mapped.

Glial cell: Non-neural immune cells and supportive cells in the brain. These support cells in the brain grey matter. They help with energy, feeding, cleansing, and protecting the neurons.

Grey matter: The neuronal portions of the brain.

Interleukins: Another type of protein or cytokine in the brain.

Karyotype: Analysis of the number and type of chromosomes in an individual. If a male patient has 46 XY then he has a normal karyotype.

Landau-Kleffner syndrome: Childhood epilepsy syndrome with normal initial language and social skills, showing loss of receptive and expressive language due to epilepsy in sleep of continuous type. Associated with abnormal sleep continuous spikes on EEG in classic cases. Variants may exist.

Lesch-Nyham syndrome: A genetically inherited disease with mental retardation, speech delay, and self-mutilation behaviors, such as biting hands, arms, and lips, or hitting oneself. Blood tests show elevated serum uric acid levels.

Limbic system: Emotional center in the brain.

Locus: This refers to one spot on a chromosome or piece of chromosome (plural: loci).

Lumbar puncture (spinal tap): Procedure to obtain cerebrospinal fluid (CSF) from the body for study from the lumbosacral spinal region under sterile technique by inserting a special needle to withdraw the CSF in a space between the posterior vertebral bodies or interspace.

Macrocephaly: Large head size.

Macrophage chemoattractant protein (MCP): Produced to attract macrophages as a result of inflammation.

Magnetic encephalography (MEG): A technique that looks at EEG-type physiology with structural images as well, to give a functional and physiological image to the brain. This uses magnetic changes in the electrical signals of the brain to provide the images. Seizure activity and functional activity can be studied.

Microcephaly: Small head size.

Mitochondria: Energy centers of the cell that when defective can be associated with brain and muscle disease that may mimic PDD and even be potentially fatal. Associated with elevated lactic acid and also may need genetic or muscle biopsy testing to diagnose.

MRI (magnetic resonance imaging): A technique for imaging the brain which uses magnetic fields to spin electrons in body tissues to give an image.

Myelin: White matter that insulates nerve fiber tracts.

Myelin basic protein: Abnormal elevated protein in CSF when damage to white matter occurs.

Naltrexone: Opioid blocking agent, may modulate pain receptors, may modulate immune system in low dose. No controlled studies yet.

Neuroglial: Glial cells in the central nervous system.

Neuron: Brain cell that performs nerve cell functions in the brain or spinal cord.

Neurotransmitter: Brain chemicals that act as messengers that transmit or activate a neuronal action in the central or peripheral nervous system.

NMDA (N-methyl-D-aspartate) receptors: Play a role in neuronal development, found on neurons and glial cells, and in areas that affect epilepsy and neuronal migration. They also play a role in modulating inflammation and cell damage by regulating glutamate influx during inflammation. They are the sites of action of drugs like memantine (Namenda).

Norepinephrine: Chemical that acts to help attention and impulsive behavior; excess helps activate flight or fight.

Open label study: Patients studied with a drug are given a medicine knowing what they are taking and the treating doctor also knows. May give preliminary results, but may be biased by placebo or desired outcome effects with better than expected results occurring.

Operculum: Region important in oral motor and emotional connections of the brain.

Opioids: Drugs that bind opiate receptors; natural opioids are enkephalins and endorphins. May play a role in pain modulation and also the immune system.

Organic acids: Acidic byproducts of chemical reactions in the body for energy metabolism. If abnormally high due to defects, may cause disease. Lactic academia, hyperglycinemia are examples.

Parietal lobes: Posterior regions associated with sensory cortex.

Pervasive developmental disorder (PDD): Part of the autistic spectrum that does not quite meet the criteria for full autism.

PET (positron emission tomography): An imaging technique that shows glucose, oxygen, or other chemical metabolism in the brain that can reveal damaged or func tional changes.

Placebo control: A patient would take an inert substance instead of active drug to see if an imagined or real treatment effect occurs.

Plagiocephaly: Flattened portion of the skull in abnormal fashion.

Quantitative EEG (QEEG): This makes quantitative EEG measurements of various frequencies and ratios of the brain waves that may detect areas of abnormal function. This is not always accepted as accurate in clinical applications.

Rett's syndrome: Known autistic spectrum disease mentioned in the DSM but now known to occur in females due to defective gene on the X-chromosome in MECP2 region.

RNA (ribonucleic acid): The matter copied from DNA in the cell nucleus or other sites that then lead to protein or other cell components being made.

Scintillation perfusion computerized tomography (SPECT): Measures blood flow and therefore crudely shows metabolism or areas of increased or decreased metabolism or relative blood flow. This can also show areas of microvascular blood flow changes when there are inflammatory changes in the brain.

Serotonin (5-hydroxytryptophan): A neurotransmitter associated with obsessive-compulsive disorder, anxiety, and depression, lack of sleep, and appetite problems when low or lacking.

Smith-Lemli-Opitz syndrome: Genetic disorder with low cholesterol levels and autistic features, with certain dysmorphic facial features and usually subnormal mental ability.

Sotos syndrome: Large head, abnormal EEG and seizures, subnormal mental development, and some atypical facial features. Genetic testing now available. Frontal prominent forehead (frontal bossing) and anti-mongoloid slant to eyes are typical.

Speech area: Regions of the brain comprising cortex that is responsible for the production of speech function either receptively or expressively: includes Wernicke's, Broca's, the opercular, motor strip, and interconnecting cortex in total, usually in the dominant hemisphere.

SSRIs (selective serotonin reuptake inhibitors): Drugs that inhibit the metabolic recycling of serotonin at the post-synaptic region of the cell junction. These are used to increase serotonin in depression, anxiety, obsessive-compulsive disorders, among other disorders. Types of SSRI include Prozac (fluoxetine), Zoloft (sertraline), Luvox (fluvoxamine), Paxil (paroxetine), Celexa (citralopram), and Lexapro (escitralopram).

Temporal lobes: Have lateral and mesial portions. Speech function is more anterior for expressive, and posterior for receptive and hearing function. Mesial sections anteriorly control memory and more posteriorly connect to emotional centers.

Translocation: Moving of a piece of chromosome from its normal position to another site, even another chromosome. This can be balanced where two pieces of genetic material trade spots, or not balanced where unequal pieces are moved to another site than normal. May or may not be associated with diseases.

Tumor necrosis factor: A protein produced as a result of inflammation by white blood cells and macrophages after cytokine reactions. Also stimulates cytokine reactions like increased IL-6 production.

Wernicke's area: Receptive speech area in the posterior temporal parietal region.

White matter: The myelinated interconnecting fiber tracts of the brain consist of white matter, non-neuronal tracts.

Williams syndrome: Genetic disorder with unusual patterns of speech and more social development than typical autism. Thought to have cerebellar-impaired mechanisms of learning. May have abnormally high calcium levels and metabolism and aortic and heart defects. Also short stature with "elfin facial features" help differentiate this from typical autism.

X-linked: Diseases associated with the X-chromosome.

Appendix 3

Resources

Books

American Psychiatric Association (1994) *Diagnostic and Statistical Manual of Mental Disorders* (4th edition, text revision). Washington, DC: American Psychiatric Association.

Attwood, T. (1998) *Asperger's Syndrome: A Guide for Parents and Professionals.* London: Jessica Kingsley Publishers.

Bauman, M.L. and Kemper, T.L. (eds) (1994) *Neurobiology of Autism.* Baltimore, MD: Johns Hopkins University Press.

Chez, M.G. (ed) (2004) 'Autism and autism spectrum disorders.' *Seminars in Pediatric Neurology 11,* 3, 185–235.

Committee on Educational Interventions for Children with Autism (2001) *National Research Council: Educating Children with Autism.* Washington, DC: National Academy Press.

Gillberg, C. and Coleman, M. (1992) *The Biology of the Autistic Syndromes* (2nd edition). London: Mac Keith Press.

Greenspan, S.I. and Wieder, S. (2006) *Engaging Autism: The Floortime Approach to Helping Children Relate, Communicate, and Think.* Reading, MA: Perseus Books.

Powers, M.D. (1989) *Children with Autism: A Parents Guide.* Bethesda, MD: Woodbine House.

Siegel, B. (1996) *The World of the Autistic Child: Understanding and Treating Autistic Spectrum Disorders.* New York: Oxford University Press.

Volkmar, F. and Wiener, L.A. (2004) *Healthcare for Children on the Autism Spectrum: A Guide to Medical, Nutritional, and Behavioral Issues.* Bethesda, MD: Woodbine House.

World Health Organization (1992) *The ICD-10 Classification of Mental and Behavioral Disorders: Clinical Descriptions and Diagnostic Guidelines.* Geneva: WHO.

Important clinical evaluation guidelines

American Academy of Pediatrics (2001) 'The pediatrician's role in the diagnosis and management of autistic spectrum disorder in children.' *Pediatrics 107*, 1221–1226.

Aman, M.G., Novotny, S., Samango-Sprouse, C., *et al.* (2004) 'Outcome measures for clinical drug trials in autism.' *CNS Spectrum 9*, 36–47.

CAN Consensus Group (1998) 'Autism screening and diagnostic evaluation: CAN consensus statement.' *CNS Spectrum 3*, 40–49.

Filipek, P.A., Accardo, P.J., Ashwal, S., *et al.* (2000) 'Practice parameter: Screening and diagnosis of autism.' Report of the Quality Standards Subcommittee of the American Academy of Neurology and Child Neurology Society. *Neurology 55*, 469–479.

Lord, C., Risi, S., Lambrecht, L., *et al.* (2000) 'The Autism Diagnostic Schedule-Generic: A standard measure of social and communication deficits associated with the spectrum of autism.' *Journal of Autism Developmental Disorders 30*, 205–223.

Lord, C., Storoschuk, S., Rutter, M., *et al.* (1993) 'Using the ADI-R to diagnose autism in preschool children.' *Infant Mental Health Journal 14*, 234–252.

Schopfler, E., Reichler, R.J., and Renner, B.R. (1998) *The Childhood Autism Rating Scale (CARS) for Diagnostic Screening and Classification in Autism.* Los Angeles, CA: Western Psychological Services.

Spence, S., Sharifi, P., and Wiznitzer, M. (2004) 'Autism spectrum disorder: Screening, diagnosis, and medical evaluation.' *Seminars in Pediatric Neurology 11*, 186–195.

South, M., Williams, B.J., McMahon, W.M., *et al.* (2002) 'Utility of the Gilliam Autism Rating Scale in research and clinical population.' *Journal of Autism and Developmental Disorders 32*, 593–599.

Volkmar, F., Cook, E.H., Pomeroy, J., *et al.* (1999) 'Practice parameters for the assessment and treatment of children and adults with autism and other pervasive developmental disorders.' American Academy of Child and Adolescent Psychiatry Working Group on Quality Issues. *Journal of the American Academy of Child and Adolescent Psychiatry 38*, 32S–54S.

World Health Organization (1993) *The ICD-10 Classification of Mental and Behavioral Disorders: Diagnostic Criteria for Research.* Geneva: WHO.

Internet and public resources

I have chosen to list those resources that support good scientific approaches to autism or offer good resource support for parents and families. There are over

57,000 autism-related sites currently on the internet search engines. This list offers credible scientific information, and may represent only a portion of informative sites available.

United States

Autism Society of America
7910 Woodmont Ave, Ste 300
Bethesda, MD 20814
301–657–0881; 800–328–8476
www.autism-society.org
National resource with local state chapters under the umbrella as well.

National Institutes of Health Autism Research Network
Bethesda, MD 20892
www.autismresearchnetwork.org
There is also an extensive listing of sites under www.nih.gov with multiple sites for autism in the various branches.
www.nimh.nih.gov/healthinformation/autismmenu.cfm

Centers for Disease Control and Prevention
1600 Clifton Rd.
Atlanta, GA 30333
800–311–3435
www.cdc.gov
www.cdc.gov/od/science/iso/concerns/mmr_autism_factsheet.htm (for information on the MMR vaccine and autism)

Organization for Autism Research (OAR)
www.researchautism.org
This is another excellent research support charity and information source for both physicians and parents.

Autism Speaks
2 Park Ave, 11th Floor
New York, NY 10016
212–252–8676
www.autismspeaks.org
This site is a great resource of information and links to research, national organizations, and also physicians. This is one of the unifying autism resource sites.

Southwest Autism Research and Resource Center (SARRC)
300 N 18th St.

Phoenix, AZ 85006
602–340–8717
www.autismcenter.org

Interdisciplinary Council on Developmental and Learning Disorders (ICDL)
4938 Hampton Lane, Ste 800
Bethesda, MD 20814
301–656–2667
www.icdl.com
Stanley Greenspan's organization for autistic spectrum and educational treatment suggestions for behavioral programs.

Treatment and Education of Autistic and Related Communication Handicapped Children (TEACCH)
www.teacch.com

American Academy of Pediatrics
www.aap.org

American Academy of Child and Adolescent Psychiatry
www.aacap.org

Child Neurology Society
www.childneurologysociety.org

National Fragile X Foundation
www.nfxf.org

International Rett Syndrome Association
www.rettsyndrome.org

Online Asperger's Syndrome Information and Support (O.A.S.I.S.)
www.aspergersyndrome.org

Charity foundations

LADDERS: Massachusetts General Program for research in autism under Margaret Bauman. www.ladders.org

Doug Flutie Jr. Foundation: Football player with autistic son started charity. www.dougflutie.org

Dan Marino Foundation: Serving greater Miami and other places as well, started by famous quarterback Dan Marino. www.danmarinofoundation.org

Canada

Autism Society of Canada
P.O. Box 635
Fredericton, New Brunswick
Canada E3B 5B4
506–363–8815
www.autismsocietycanada.ca

United Kingdom

National Autistic Society
393 City Rd
London EC1V 1NG
020 7833 2299
www.nas.org.uk

Friends of Landau-Kleffner (FOLKS)
www.friendsoflks.com

Autism Awareness
www.autism-awareness.org.uk

Australia

Australian Advisory Board on Autism Spectrum Disorders
www.autismaus.com.au

Autism Victoria
www.autismvictoria.org.au

Statewide Autistic Services
www.sasi.org.au

Asperger Services Australia
www.asperger.asn.au

Index